THIS KETO PLANNER

BELONGS TO:

____

GOALS

WHEN	MY GOALS	STEPS
6 MONTHS		
1 YEAR		
2 YEARS		
5 YEARS		

INSPIRATION

GOALS

Now focus on goals that have nothing to do with weight.
You are so much more than what you weigh.

WHEN	MY GOALS	STEPS
6 MONTHS		
1 YEAR		
2 YEARS		
5 YEARS		

INSPIRATION

START POINT

DATE:

	MEASUREMENT:	GOAL:
WEIGHT:		
LEFT ARM:		
RIGHT ARM:		
CHEST:		
WAIST:		
HIPS:		
LEFT THIGH:		
RIGHT THIGH:		

Weekly Goals

EXERCISE: 12 WEEKS

1 Rest	2 Upper Body	3 Cardio	4 Abs	5 Cardio	6 Lower Body	7 Cardio
8 Rest	9 Upper Body	10 Cardio	11 Abs	12 Cardio	13 Lower Body	14 Cardio
15 Rest	16 Upper Body	17 Cardio	18 Abs	19 Cardio	20 Lower Body	21 Cardio
22 Rest	23 Upper Body	24 Cardio	25 Abs	26 Cardio	27 Lower Body	28 Cardio
29 Rest	30 Upper Body	31 Cardio	32 Abs	33 Cardio	34 Lower Body	35 Cardio
36 Rest	37 Upper Body	38 Cardio	39 Abs	40 Cardio	41 Lower Body	42 Cardio
43 Rest	44 Upper Body	45 Cardio HIIT	46 Abs	47 Cardio HIIT	48 Lower Body HIIT	49 Cardio
50 Rest	51 Upper Body	52 Cardio HIIT	53 Abs	54 Cardio HIIT	55 Lower Body HIIT	56 Cardio
57 Rest	58 Upper Body	59 Cardio HIIT	60 Abs	61 Cardio HIIT	62 Lower Body HIIT	63 Cardio
64 Rest	65 Upper Body	66 Cardio HIIT	67 Abs	68 Cardio HIIT	69 Lower Body HIIT	70 Cardio
71 Rest	72 Upper Body	73 Cardio HIIT	74 Abs	75 Cardio HIIT	76 Lower Body HIIT	77 Cardio
78 Rest	79 Upper Body	80 Cardio HIIT	81 Abs	82 Cardio HIIT	83 Lower Body HIIT	84 Cardio

WEEK 1 WORKOUTS

These ideas are free and can be done anywhere, but the best exercise is something you enjoy! Try a new class, active hobby, or video for fun.

MON	**Recovery Day:** *gentle yoga, stretching* **Choose a recovery day that works best for your schedule**
TUE	**Upper Body:** *Walk 10 minutes, 10 pushups 10 tricep dips on a bench or chair 10 supermans*
WED	**Cardio:** *Walk 5 minutes, Run/Jog 5 minutes Walk 5 minutes*
THUR	**Abs:** *Walk 5 minutes, 50 crunches. Hold plank 1 minute* **(modification on knees),** *hold boat pose 30 seconds*
FRI	**Cardio:** *Walk 5 minutes, Run/Jog 5 minutes Walk 5 minutes*. **If possible, use stairs or jog on an incline to work different muscle groups.**
SAT	**Lower Body:** *Walk 5 minutes, 50 squats, 50 lunges, 1 minute wall sit*
SUN	**Cardio:** *Walk, hike, bike, swim or dance 30 minutes.* **Push yourself a little farther today. You get to rest tomorrow!**

WEEK 2 WORKOUTS

This week has a few longer workout sessions. If that works for you, great! If you just don't have the time, do a shorter workout.

MON	**Recovery Day:** *gentle yoga, stretching* **Choose a recovery day that works best for your schedule**
TUE	**Upper Body:** *Walk 15 minutes, 15 pushups, 15 tricep dips on a bench or chair, 15 supermans*
WED	**Cardio:** *Walk 5 minutes, Run/Jog 10 minutes, Walk 5 minutes*
THUR	**Abs:** *Walk 5 minutes, 150 crunches. Hold plank 1:30 minutes.*
FRI	**Cardio:** *Walk 5 minutes, Run/Jog 10 minutes Walk 5 minutes.* **If possible, use stairs or jog on an incline to work different muscle groups.**
SAT	**Lower Body:** *Walk 10 minutes, 100 squats, 100 lunges, 1:30 minute wall sit*
SUN	**Cardio:** *Walk, hike, bike, swim or dance 40 minutes.* **Push yourself a little farther today. You get to rest tomorrow!**

WEEK 3 WORKOUTS

You are getting stronger every day! Stay motivated and don't forget self-care. Consider starting a short meditation routine each morning.

MON	**Recovery Day:** *gentle yoga, stretching* **Choose a recovery day that works best for your schedule**
TUE	**Upper Body:** *Walk 20 minutes, 20 pushups, 20 tricep dips on a bench or chair, 20 supermans*
WED	**Cardio:** *Walk 5 minutes, Run/Jog 15 minutes, Walk 5 minutes*
THUR	**Abs:** *Walk 5 minutes, 200 crunches. Hold plank 2 minutes.*
FRI	**Cardio:** *Walk 5 minutes, Run/Jog 15 minutes Walk 5 minutes.* **If possible, use stairs or jog on an incline to work different muscle groups.**
SAT	**Lower Body:** *Walk 15 minutes, 150 squats, 150 lunges, 2 minute wall sit*
SUN	**Cardio:** *Walk, hike, bike, swim or dance 30 minutes.* **Push yourself a little farther today. You get to rest tomorrow!**

WEEK 4 WORKOUTS

This week we add weights. If you have dumbbells, great! If not, use soup cans or bottled water. Start light (especially for shoulders).

MON	**Recovery Day:** *gentle yoga, stretching* **Choose a recovery day that works best for your schedule**
TUE	**Upper Body:** *Walk 30 minutes, 20 pushups, 20 tricep dips on a bench or chair, 20 supermans, 20 bicep curls + 20 shoulder presses with weights*
WED	**Cardio:** *Walk 5 minutes, Run/Jog 25 minutes, Walk 5 minutes*
THUR	**Abs:** *Walk 10 minutes, 200 crunches. Hold plank 3 minutes.*
FRI	**Cardio:** *Walk 5 minutes, Run/Jog 20 minutes Walk 5 minutes.* **If possible, use stairs or jog on an incline to work different muscle groups.**
SAT	**Lower Body:** *Walk 15 minutes, 150 squats, 150 lunges, 2 minute wall sit 50 squats + 50 lunges with weights*
SUN	**Cardio:** *Walk, hike, bike, swim or dance 60 minutes.* **Push yourself a little farther today. You get to rest tomorrow!**

WEEK 5 WORKOUTS

If you are up for a challenge, try a higher weight for your last 10 sets of bicep curls, squats and lunges.

MON	**Recovery Day:** *gentle yoga, stretching* **Choose a recovery day that works best for your schedule**
TUE	**Upper Body:** *Walk 30 minutes, 30 pushups, 30 tricep dips on a bench or chair, 30 supermans, 30 bicep curls + 30 shoulder presses with weights*
WED	**Cardio:** *Walk 5 minutes, Run/Jog 35 minutes, Walk 5 minutes*
THUR	**Abs:** *Walk 10 minutes, 200 crunches. Hold plank 3 minutes.*
FRI	**Cardio:** *Walk 5 minutes, Run/Jog 25 minutes Walk 5 minutes.* **If possible, use stairs or jog on an incline to work different muscle groups.**
SAT	**Lower Body:** *Walk 15 minutes, 150 squats, 150 lunges, 3 minute wall sit 100 squats + 100 lunges with weights*
SUN	**Cardio:** *Walk, hike, bike, swim or dance 60 minutes.* **Push yourself a little farther today. You get to rest tomorrow!**

WEEK 6 WORKOUTS

You are half-way there! The workouts get longer and more intense each week, but do what works best for you. This is about feeling good.

MON	**Recovery Day:** *gentle yoga, stretching* **Choose a recovery day that works best for your schedule**
TUE	**Upper Body:** *Walk 30 minutes, 30 pushups, 30 tricep dips on a bench or chair, 30 supermans, 30 bicep curls + 30 shoulder presses + 30 chest presses with weights*
WED	**Cardio:** *Walk 5 minutes, Run/Jog 40 minutes, Walk 5 minutes*
THUR	**Abs:** *Walk 10 minutes, 200 crunches. Hold plank 3 minutes.*
FRI	**Cardio:** *Walk 5 minutes, Run/Jog 30 minutes Walk 5 minutes.* **If possible, use stairs or jog on an incline to work different muscle groups.**
SAT	**Lower Body:** *Walk 15 minutes, 150 squats, 150 lunges, 3 minute wall sit, 100 squats + 100 lunges + 100 calf raises with weights*
SUN	**Cardio:** *Jog, hike, bike, swim or dance 60 minutes.* **Push yourself a little farther today. You get to rest tomorrow!**

WEEK 7 WORKOUTS

These workouts begin to incorporate High Intensity Interval Training (HIIT) to boost your metabolism.

MON	**Recovery Day:** *gentle yoga, stretching* **Choose a recovery day that works best for your schedule**
TUE	**Upper Body:** *Walk 30 minutes, 30 pushups, 30 tricep dips on a bench or chair, 30 supermans, 30 bicep curls + 30 shoulder presses + 30 chest presses with weights*
WED	**Cardio HIIT:** *Walk 5 minutes, Sprint 1 minute Run/Jog 10 minutes Sprint 1 minute Run/Jog 10 minutes Walk 5 minutes*
THUR	**Abs:** *Walk 10 minutes, 200 crunches. Hold plank 3 minutes. Hold boat pose 1 minute*
FRI	**Cardio:** *Walk 5 minutes, Run/Jog 35 minutes Walk 5 minutes.* **If possible, use stairs or jog on an incline to work different muscle groups.**
SAT	**Lower Body HIIT:** *Walk 15 minutes, 50 jumping squats, 50 jumping lunges, 3 minute wall sit. 150 squats + 150 lunges with weights*
SUN	**Cardio:** *Jog, hike, bike, swim or dance 60 minutes.* **Push yourself a little farther today. You get to rest tomorrow!**

WEEK 8 WORKOUTS

You have been at this almost two months! Good work. Keep focused.

MON	**Recovery Day:** *gentle yoga, stretching* Choose a recovery day that works best for your schedule
TUE	**Upper Body:** *Walk 30 minutes, 30 pushups, 30 tricep dips on a bench or chair, 30 bicep curls + 30 shoulder presses + 30 chest presses with weights*
WED	**Cardio HIIT:** *Walk 5 minutes, Sprint 1 minute Run/Jog 10 minutes Sprint 1 minute Run/Jog 10 minutes Sprint 1 minute Run/Jog 10 minutes Walk 5 minutes*
THUR	**Abs:** *Walk 15 minutes, Hold boat pose 2 minutes Hold plank 3 minutes.*
FRI	**Cardio:** *Walk 5 minutes, Run/Jog 35 minutes Sprint 2 minutes Walk 5 minutes.* If possible, use stairs or jog on an incline to work different muscle groups.
SAT	**Lower Body HIIT:** *Walk 5 minutes, 100 jumping squats, 100 jumping lunges, 3 minute wall sit. 150 squats + 150 lunges with weights*
SUN	**Cardio:** *Run, hike, bike, swim or dance 60 minutes.* Push yourself a little farther today. You get to rest tomorrow!

WEEK 9 WORKOUTS

Consider increasing your weights. Challenge yourself. If the longer runs are too time consuming, lower your jogging time and increase your sprints.

MON	**Recovery Day:** *gentle yoga, stretching* **Choose a recovery day that works best for your schedule**
TUE	**Upper Body:** *Walk 30 minutes, 30 pushups, 30 chest presses. 30 bicep curls, 30 shoulder presses + 30 chest presses with weights*
WED	**Cardio HIIT:** *Walk 5 minutes, Sprint 1 minute Run/Jog 10 minutes Sprint 1 minute Run/Jog 10 minutes Sprint 1 minute Run/Jog 10 minutes Walk 5 minutes*
THUR	**Abs:** *Walk 15 minutes, Hold boat pose 3 minutes Hold plank 3 minutes.*
FRI	**Cardio:** *Walk 5 minutes, Run/Jog 35 minutes Sprint 3 minutes Walk 5 minutes. If possible, use stairs or go on an incline.*
SAT	**Lower Body HIIT:** *Walk 15 minutes, 120 jumping squats, 120 jumping lunges, 3 minute wall sit. 150 squats + 150 lunges with weights*
SUN	**Cardio:** *Run, hike, bike, swim or dance 60 minutes.* **Push yourself a little farther today. You get to rest tomorrow!**

WEEK 10 WORKOUTS

You are doing great! Keep up your motivation. Swap out a workout for an online HIIT video if you need some guidance.

MON	**Recovery Day:** *gentle yoga, stretching* **Choose a recovery day that works best for your schedule**
TUE	**Upper Body:** *Walk 30 minutes, 30 pushups, 30 chest presses, 30 bicep curls, 30 shoulder presses + 30 chest presses with weights*
WED	**Cardio HIIT:** *Walk 5 minutes, Sprint 1 minute Run/Jog 10 minutes Sprint 1 minute Run/Jog 10 minutes Sprint 2 minutes Run/Jog 10 minutes Sprint 3 minutes Walk 5 minutes*
THUR	**Abs:** *Walk 30 minutes, Hold boat pose 3 minutes Hold plank 3 minutes, 100 crunches.*
FRI	**Cardio:** *Walk 5 minutes, Run/Jog 35 minutes Sprint 3 minutes Walk 5 minutes.* **If possible, use stairs or go on an incline to work different muscle groups.**
SAT	**Lower Body HIIT:** *Walk 15 minutes, 150 jumping squats, 150 jumping lunges, 3 minute wall sit, 150 squats, 150 lunges, 150 calf raises with weights*
SUN	**Cardio:** *Run, hike, bike, swim or dance 60 minutes.* **Push yourself a little farther today. You get to rest tomorrow!**

WEEK 11 WORKOUTS

Watch your self talk this week. Talk to yourself the way you would to a friend. Be proud of your accomplishments.

MON	**Recovery Day:** gentle yoga, stretching **Choose a recovery day that works best for your schedule**
TUE	**Upper Body:** Walk 30 minutes, 30 pushups, 30 chest presses. 30 bicep curls, 30 shoulder presses + 30 chest presses with weights
WED	**Cardio HIIT:** Walk 5 minutes, Sprint 1 minute Run/Jog 10 minutes Sprint 1 minute Run/Jog 10 minutes Sprint 2 minutes Run/Jog 10 minutes Sprint 3 minutes Walk 5 minutes
THUR	**Abs:** Walk 30 minutes, Hold boat pose 3 minutes Hold plank 3 minutes. 100 crunches.
FRI	**Cardio:** Walk 5 minutes, Run/Jog 35 minutes Sprint 3 minutes Walk 5 minutes. If possible, use stairs or go on an incline.
SAT	**Lower Body HIIT:** Walk 15 minutes, 5 burpees, 150 jumping squats, 150 jumping lunges, 3 minute wall sit. 150 squats + 150 lunges + 150 calf raises with weights
SUN	**Cardio:** Run, hike, bike, swim or dance 60 minutes. **Push yourself a little farther today. You get to rest tomorrow!**

WEEK 12 WORKOUTS

It's the last week of this journal, but not the last week that you work out. Commit yourself to taking care of your body and mind. Congratulations!

MON	**Recovery Day:** *gentle yoga, stretching* **Choose a recovery day that works best for your schedule**
TUE	**Upper Body:** *Walk 30 minutes, 30 pushups, 30 chest presses. 30 bicep curls, 30 shoulder presses + 30 chest presses with weights*
WED	**Cardio HIIT:** *Walk 5 minutes, Sprint 2 minutes Run/Jog 10 minutes Sprint 1 minute Run/Jog 10 minutes Sprint 2 minutes Run/Jog 10 minutes Sprint 3 minutes Walk 5 minutes*
THUR	**Abs:** *Walk 30 minutes, Hold boat pose 3 minutes Hold plank 3 minutes. 100 twisting crunches.*
FRI	**Cardio:** *Walk 5 minutes, Run/Jog 35 minutes Sprint 3 minutes Walk 5 minutes.* **If possible, use stairs or jog on an incline to work different muscle groups.**
SAT	**Lower Body HIIT:** *Walk 15 minutes, 10 burpees, 150 jumping squats, 150 jumping lunges, 3 minute wall sit. 150 squats + 150 lunges + 150 calf raises with weights*
SUN	**Cardio:** *Run, hike, bike, swim or dance 60 minutes.* **Push yourself a little farther today. You get to rest tomorrow!**

WEEK 1 MEAL PLANS

	BREAKFAST	LUNCH	DINNER
MON	Butter Coffee, Avocado Eggs with salsa and bacon	Turkey wrap with Green smoothie	Broiled salmon with zucchini noodles + Alfredo sauce with buttered asparagus
TUES	Scrambled eggs with cheese and sausage	Salmon Nicoise Salad	Slow cooker shredded pork with salad and roasted cauliflower
WED	Raspberry smoothie	Roast beef/cheese roll up + mayo and horseradish 1/2 green apple	Ginger Steak and Bok Choy Stir-fry
THU	Egg muffins	Bunless bacon cheeseburger with blue cheese and mushrooms	Meatballs + zucchini noodles with spaghetti sauce + cheese, steamed broccoli with butter
FRI	Chia pudding with berries	Buffalo chicken wings with celery + blue cheese dressing	Chili + salad
SAT	Plain Greek yogurt + keto blueberry syrup	Grilled cheese with leftover chili & cheese + salad	Chicken curry with zucchini + bell pepper on cauliflower rice
SUN	Cheesy omelet + bell pepper and ham	Portobello pizza	Pot Roast with roasted cauliflower

WEEK 1 MEAL PLANS

DAY 1

BREAKFAST:

Butter Coffee blend hot coffee with 1 tbsp each butter + melted coconut oil. *Avocado Eggs with salsa and bacon* Cut **avocado** in ½ and remove pit. Scoop out about 1 tbsp of avocado on each side. Crack **egg** into avocado. Microwave for 1-2 minutes in 30 second bursts until cooked. Can also bake in baking dish at 425° F for 15 minutes. Serve with salsa and bacon and fresh avocado.

LUNCH:

Turkey wrap **Turkey, bacon, cheese, mayo** wrapped in romaine **lettuce**
Green smoothie In blender, pulse 1 can full fat coconut milk or 1 cup full fat **Greek yogurt**, 1 tsp **vanilla extract**, 1 cup **spinach** with ½ cup **frozen berries.**

DINNER:

Broiled salmon with zucchini noodles + Alfredo sauce with buttered asparagus Broil **salmon** sprinkled with lemon pepper for 15 minutes. Line pan with aluminum foil for easy clean up. Sauté **zucchini noodles** in ½ tbsp oil until cooked through. Alfredo: melt 2 tbsp **butte**r and 3 oz **cream cheese** in a pot over low heat, whisking to combine. Add 1/2 cup of **heavy cream** and 1/2 cup of **parmesan cheese** until melted. Or buy bottled full fat Alfredo and check label for lower carbs.

SNACKS:

Microwave keto bread: Mix 3 tbsp blanched **almond flour** with ½ tsp **baking powder**. Stir in 1 tbsp melted **butter** and 1 **egg**. Pour into mug or ramekin. Microwave for 90 seconds. Let cool for a few minutes. Can also bake in oven preheated to 375° F for 10 minutes.

1/4 cup almonds + 2 squares dark chocolate

WATER INTAKE:

WEEK 1 MEAL PLANS

DAY 2

BREAKFAST:

Scrambled eggs with cheese and sausage sandwich Melt butter in pan. Add beaten **eggs** and cook. Sprinkle with **cheese** and serve with **sausage** or bacon on *Keto bread* Mix 3 tbsp blanched **almond flour** with ½ tsp **baking powder**. Stir in 1 tbsp melted **butter** and 1 **egg**. Pour into mug or ramekin. Microwave for 90 seconds. Let cool for a few minutes. Or bake in oven at 375° F for 10 minutes. *Coffee with heavy cream*

LUNCH:

Keto Nicoise Salad with leftover salmon Cut leftover **salmon** (or **canned tuna**) and two **hard boiled eggs** into bite-sized chunks. Combine with ½ cup steamed or microwaved **green beans** and sliced **black olives**. Stir in two tbsp of **Greek yogurt** and a tsp of **red wine vinegar**. Salt & pepper to taste. Good hot or cold.

DINNER:

Slow cooker shredded pork with salad and roasted cauliflower Place **pork loin** in crock pot with 1 cup **salsa** and cook on low for 8-12 hours. Serve with sour cream, avocado, salsa.
Roast chopped **cauliflower** with olive oil at 425° F for 15-20 minutes.
Line pan with aluminum foil for easy clean up.

SNACKS:

Avocado with salt and lime juice

Apple slices with almond butter

WATER INTAKE: ☐ ☐ ☐ ☐ ☐ ☐ ☐ ☐

WEEK 1 MEAL PLANS

DAY 3

BREAKFAST:

Raspberry smoothie

Blend together 1 cup plain full fat **Greek Yogurt**, 1/2 cup **heavy cream** or plain almond milk, 1 scoop **protein powder**, 1/2 cup **frozen raspberrie**s and 2-4 drops liquid stevia (or to taste) in blender until mixed thoroughly. Add water to thin if consistency is too thick.

LUNCH:

Roast beef/cheese roll up + mayo and horseradish to taste with 1/2 green apple

DINNER:

Broccoli Beef Stir Fry Cut two **steaks** into tiny slices. Heat in non stick pan with sesame oil. While beef is cooking, combine 4 tbsp **soy sauce**, 2 **tbsp sesame oil**, ½ tbsp **ginger paste**, and 2-4 tsp **Yuzu sauce**. Microwave 2 cups **broccoli** pieces in microwave for 1 minute and then add to pan (you can also add raw broccoli to pan with beef and add a little beef broth or water and let steam for 2 minutes with cover). Cook for 2 minutes. Add **Yuzu sesame mixture**, heat and serve.

SNACKS:

Berries with heavy cream

Macadamia Nuts

WATER INTAKE:

WEEK 1 MEAL PLANS

DAY 4

BREAKFAST:

Egg muffins Preheat oven to 350° F. Whisk 12 **eggs** in a bowl. Spray a 12 capacity muffin tin with oil. Fill each tin with **diced ham** (or bacon or sausage) and chopped **red pepper**. Pour whisked egg mixture over each tin to fill about 2/3 full. Top each tin with **shredded cheese**. Bake for 15 minutes or until set. Let cool and serve. You can freeze these for a quick and easy breakfast later.

LUNCH:

Bunless bacon cheeseburger with blue cheese and mushrooms sautéed in butter

DINNER:

Italian Meatballs on zucchini noodles with salad Mix 1/2 lb **ground beef** with 1/2 lb **ground pork** with one **egg**, 1 tsp **salt** and 2 tsp **Italian seasoning** in a bowl and combine thoroughly. Form into small balls. Heat olive oil in a large pan and sauté the meatballs until golden brown and cooked through. Lower heat and add 14 oz can of **crushed tomatoes** or low carb spaghetti sauce. Simmer for 15 minutes, stirring occasionally. Season with salt & pepper. Meanwhile, heat 1/2 tbsp olive oil in separate pan and sauté **zucchini noodles** until cooked through. Cover meatballs and sauce with shredded mozzarella cheese and serve with zucchini.

SNACKS:

Celery sticks with almond butter

Pork rinds (check label for added sugar)

WATER INTAKE:

WEEK 1 MEAL PLANS

DAY 5

BREAKFAST:

Coconut milk pudding with strawberries: Refrigerate full fat **coconut milk** overnight, blend until smooth and serve with **berries**.

LUNCH:

Buffalo chicken wings with celery + blue cheese dressing Combine 4 tbsp melted **butter** with 1/4 cup **hot sauce**. Dip 12 **chicken wings** in butter/hot sauce mix and salt pepper. Bake at 400° F for 45 minutes or until crispy. Serve with celery and low carb blue cheese or ranch dressing.

DINNER:

Low Carb chili and Salad For chili, sauté ½ chopped **onion** and a chopped **red bell pepper** in olive oil until soft. Add 1 lb **ground beef** and cook until no longer pink. Add 1 tbsp **chili powder**, 1 tsp **cumin**, 1/2 tbsp **cocoa power**, 1 tsp **salt** and stir. Add one 14 oz can crushed or **diced tomatoe**s and heat. Thin with broth or water if needed. Serve with sour cream and shredded cheese. Good with keto bread (see Day 1 snacks).

SNACKS:

Hardboiled eggs, cheese and nuts

Greek yogurt and berries

WATER INTAKE:

WEEK 1 MEAL PLANS

DAY 6

BREAKFAST:

Plain Greek yogurt with blueberries and no sugar maple syrup or keto blueberry syrup
For syrup, melt ¼ cup **blueberries** with 2 tbsp **butter**

LUNCH:

Grilled cheese or favorite sandwich on keto bread Mix 3 tbsp blanched **almond flour** with ½ tsp **baking powder**. Stir in 1 tbsp melted **butter** and 1 **egg**. Pour into mug or ramekin. Microwave for 90 seconds. Let cool for a few minutes. Can bake in oven preheated to 375° F for 10 minutes. *Leftover chili + salad*

DINNER:

Chicken curry with zucchini + bell pepper on cauliflower rice Cut **chicken** into bite-sized pieces and cook in coconut oil in pan. When no longer pink, add sliced **zucchini** and **bell pepper** and sauté until softened. Add one can of full fat **coconut milk** to pan with 1 tbsp green **curry paste** (or curry powder). Serve with steamed cauliflower rice.

SNACKS:

Raw red and green pepper strips with guacamole

Cream cheese with macadamia nuts

WATER INTAKE:

WEEK 1 MEAL PLANS

DAY 7

BREAKFAST:

Cheesy omelet + green bell pepper and ham

LUNCH:

Portobello pizzas Line pan with aluminum foil. Brush two clean large **Portobello mushroom caps** (stems removed) with olive oil and place on pan. Spread **pizza sauce** on inside of mushroom caps, add **pepperoni** or ham and **cheese**. Broil until cheese is melted, 6-9 minutes.

DINNER:

Pot Roast + roasted cauliflower

Place 2-4 lb **beef roast** in crock pot with 2 cups **broth**, 2 tsp salt, and 2 tbsp **Worcestershire sauce**. Add 1 cup **radishe**s cut into large pieces and one large **onion** cut into large pieces. Heat on low for 8-10 hours or high for 5-6. Serve with roasted **cauliflower**. Drizzle cauliflower with olive oil and bake at 425° F for 25 minutes. Optional: put cauliflower florets in crock pot for last 30-40 minutes.

SNACKS:

Cheddar cheese crisps with jalapenos Line a baking sheet with parchment paper. Divide 1 cup grated **cheddar cheese** into mounds (1-3 tbsp per mound) and add a thin **jalapeno slice** to each mound. Bake at 375° F for 10 minutes or until crisp. Let cool.

Sunflower seeds with clementine orange

WATER INTAKE:

WEEK 2 MEAL PLANS

	BREAKFAST	LUNCH	DINNER
MON	Veggie Frittata	Chicken Guacamole Wraps	Chicken and roasted veggies with Tahini dressing
TUES	Almond Butter Frappe	Pepperoni Pizza Cups	Slow Cooker Butter Chicken
WED	Strawberry nut smoothie	Turkey Caprese wrap	Roast chicken with steamed broccoli and butter
THU	Keto Pancakes	Tuna spinach salad	Santa Maria Tri tip with broccoli slaw
FRI	Not Oatmeal	Steak salad	Reuben Corned Beef with Sauerkraut
SAT	Cheese omelet	Cucumber Salmon "sandwiches"	Pesto Chicken with Asparagus
SUN	Huevos rancheros	Caesar Salad	Mushroom, Onion and Swiss burgers

WEEK 2 MEAL PLANS

DAY 1

BREAKFAST:

Veggie Frittata Sauté **onion** and **red pepper** in an oven proof medium skillet until soft. Add 4 beaten **eggs** into pan and tilt pan to distribute evenly. Let cook for 1-2 minutes more then bake in oven for 10-15 minutes at 350° F.

LUNCH:

Chicken Bacon Guacamole Wraps Mash 2 tbsp **lime juice** with ¼ tsp **salt** and a peeled **avocado** (or buy guacamole with no added sugar). Spread on romaine **lettuce** leaves and add shredded leftover roast **chicken** and **bacon**.

DINNER:

Chicken and roasted veggies with Tahini dressing
Roast **asparagus** and **cauliflower** drizzled with olive oil for 15-20 minutes at 425° F. Serve with shredded **chicken** and tahini lemon sauce. For sauce, mix 2 tbsp **tahini** with 1 tbsp **lemon juice** and 1 tbsp water (or more if you like a thinner sauce).

SNACKS:

Apples with cream cheese

2 squares dark chocolate and pumpkin seeds

WATER INTAKE:

WEEK 2 MEAL PLANS

DAY 2

BREAKFAST:

Almond Butter Frappe Blend together 1 cup brewed **coffee**, frozen in ice cubes, 1 tbsp **almond butter**, 1/4 cup **heavy cream**, almond milk, or coconut milk. Optional: add 3-5 drops liquid stevia.

LUNCH:

Pepperoni Pizza Cups Line muffin tin. with **pepperoni.** Bake at 400° F for 5 minutes. Remove and allow to cool for 5 minutes. Put ½-1 tsp of **tomato paste** in each cup. Cover each round in **mozzarella cheese** and Bake for 3-5 minutes until melted. *Salad with low carb dressing*

DINNER:

Slow Cooker Butter Chicken Add 3 tbsp **butte**r to a large skillet or saucepan and cook 1/2 chopped **onion** and 1 diced **garlic clove** until soft, about 5 minutes. Add 1 tbsp **cumin**, 3 tsp **garam masala**, 2 tsp **turmeric**, 1 tsp **chili powder**, 1 tsp **cinnamon** and 1 tsp **salt**. Cook for another 1-2 minutes. Transfer onion mixture to crock pot. Add two **chicken breasts** cut into bite-sized pieces, one 15 oz can full fat **coconut milk**, one 15 oz can **tomato sauce** to crock pot. Cover and cook on high for 2-3 hours or low for 6-7 hours. Add 1 cup chopped **green beans** about an hour before serving. Enjoy with steamed **cauliflower rice**.

SNACKS:

Avocado Chocolate Mousse In double boiler, melt 2 ounces of **dark chocolate**. Add 2 tbsp of **cream cheese** and combine well. Stir in 1 tsp **vanilla** & remove from heat. In bowl, smash an **avocado** with a fork. Add chocolate mix to avocado and combine. In a separate bowl, beat ¼ cup **heavy cream** until whipped. Gently stir whipped cream into avocado chocolate. Divide into four ramekins and chill in the refrigerator.

Ham and cheese

WATER INTAKE:

WEEK 2 MEAL PLANS

DAY 3

BREAKFAST:

Strawberry nut smoothie

Blend together 1 cup unsweetened **almond milk**, 1/2 cup **heavy cream**, 1 scoop **protein powder**, 1/2 cup **frozen strawberries**, 2 tbsp **almond butter** and 3-4 drops liquid s**tevia** or to taste

LUNCH:

Turkey Caprese wrap: **Turkey, mozzarella cheese, fresh basil,** and **tomato** wrapped in romaine **lettuce** Dip: 2 tbsp **olive oil** and 2 tsp **balsamic vinegar**

Greek yogurt + frozen berries

DINNER:

Roast chicken with steamed broccoli and butter

On busy days, pick up a **roast chicken** in the deli department and a bag of **broccoli** with a **salad**. Or roast a whole chicken at 450° F for 50-60 minutes. Place broccoli florets on a large sheet and drizzle with 2 tablespoons of olive oil and salt and roast for 20 minutes.

SNACKS:

Salami and string cheese

½ cup macadamia nuts + 2 squares dark chocolate

WATER INTAKE:

WEEK 2 MEAL PLANS

DAY 4

BREAKFAST:

Keto Pancakes Combine 4 oz **cream cheese** with 4 **eggs** and 4 tbsp of **coconut flour** (or 8 tbsp of almond flour), 1/8 tsp **salt**, 1/2 tsp **vanilla** and a few drops of **stevia**. Heat a skillet and melt butter in the pan. Heat on both sides and serve with no sugar syrup or **blueberries** mixed with melted **butter**.

LUNCH:

Tuna spinach salad **Spinach** salad with **hardboiled eggs**, canned **tuna**, and sliced **avocado.** For dressing, mix full fat **mayo** with **lemon juice**, salt and pepper.

DINNER:

Santa Maria Tri tip with broccoli slaw Marinate the **bee**f in 1/3 cup **red wine vinegar** and 1/3 cup **olive oil** with 1 tbsp **kosher salt**, 1 tsp **black pepper** and 1 tsp **garlic salt**. Grill and serve. You can also bake in the oven at 375° F for 45-60 minutes. For slaw, toss 2 cups shredded **broccoli** with ¼ cup **olive oil,** 1/8 cup **vinegar**, ¼ tsp **Italian seasoning**, and salt & pepper to taste. Refrigerate for several hours.

SNACKS:

Roasted seaweed strips

Beef jerky (no sugar added)

WATER INTAKE:

WEEK 2 MEAL PLANS

DAY 5

BREAKFAST:

Not Oatmeal: Mix together 2 tbsp **heavy cream**, coconut milk or almond milk with 2 tbsp water and 3 tbsp blanched **almond flour** and a dash of salt. Warm in saucepan over low heat or microwave for one minute. Serve with unsweetened coconut flakes, slivered almonds and fresh berries.

LUNCH:

Steak salad Use leftover **tri tip** sliced thin. Serve over **spinach** and **arugula mix** with shaved **Parmesan cheese**. Drizzle with 2 tbsp **olive oil** and 2 tsp **balsamic vinegar**

Blueberries with almonds

DINNER:

Reuben Corned Beef with Sauerkraut

Place 1/2 lb **shredded corn beef** in a casserole dish. In bowl, combine 2 **eggs** with ½ cup each **mayo** and **whipping cream**, ½ tsp **dry mustard** and 2/3 cup drained & rinsed **sauerkraut**. Pour mayo mix over beef and sprinkle with 2 cups shredded Swiss cheese. Bake covered for 30 minutes at 375° F . Uncover and bake for another 15 minutes.

SNACKS:

Cheese and nuts

Peanut butter and dark chocolate

WATER INTAKE:

WEEK 2 MEAL PLANS

DAY 6

BREAKFAST:

Cheese omelet with spinach

LUNCH:

Cucumber Salmon "sandwiches"
Slice one **cucumber** and spread **cream cheese** on each round. Add **smoked salmon**. Great with fresh dill.

Hardboiled egg and macadamia nuts

DINNER:

Pesto Chicken with Asparagus Pesto: Place 2 cups **arugula**, ¼ cup **olive oil**, ¼ cup toasted* **walnuts** or pine nuts, 1/4 cup **Parmesan cheese**, 1 clove **garlic** (peeled), juice of ½ **lemon** and dash of salt and pepper in food processor. Pulse until combined. Toss **chicken** in pesto and bake at 375° F for 30 minutes. *Toast walnuts at 375° F for 6 minutes and pine nuts for 8-10 minutes. Serve with steamed and buttered asparagus.

SNACKS:

Parmesan Chips: Line baking sheet with parchment paper. Put 1 tbsp of **parmesan cheese** for each "chip" and flatten. Leave space between chips. Bake at 400° F for 3-5 minutes.

Sunflower seeds

WATER INTAKE:

WEEK 2 MEAL PLANS

DAY 7

BREAKFAST:

Huevos Rancheros Fry two **egg**s in butter. Serve with **guacamole** and your favorite **salsa.**

LUNCH:

Caesar Salad **Romaine lettuce**, leftover pesto **chicken**, grated **parmesan cheese** with Caesar dressing (bottled or mix 4 tbsp **lemon juice** with ¼ cup **olive oil**, 1 /2 tsp **Worcestershire sauce**, ½ tsp salt, 1 clove of **garlic**, peeled & smashed, 1 raw **egg**, ½ cup **Parmesan cheese**, 1 tsp pepper, and squeeze of **anchovy paste**).

DINNER:

Mushroom, Onion and Swiss burgers. Grill **burgers**. Sauté **mushroom**s and **sliced onions** in butter until cooked through. Add a dash of **Worcestershire sauce** and serve over burgers with mushrooms, onions and Swiss cheese.

SNACKS:

Almonds and apple slices

Lemon fat bombs: melt 1/3 cup **coconut butter** 1/3 cup **coconut oil** on a double boiler. Add 2 tsp **lemon zest** and 2 tbsp **lemon juice**. Freeze in silicone muffin mold until set. Keep in airtight container in the refrigerator.

WATER INTAKE:

WEEK 3 MEAL PLANS

	BREAKFAST	LUNCH	DINNER
MON	Cloud bread	Cobb Salad	Cauliflower Bacon Bake
TUES	Eggs Benedict with hollandaise sauce	Cloud Bread Pizza	Slow Swedish Meatballs with cabbage pasta
WED	Chia seed coconut pudding with raspberries	Salmon Cakes with Lemon Butter Sauce	Ensenada chicken & Salad
THU	Scrambled eggs with sausage	Fajita Bowl	Gyoza Filling Wraps
FRI	Chocolate Peanut Butter Smoothie	Goat Cheese salad	Greek Chicken Bake
SAT	Fried eggs with spinach sautéed in butter	Italian Wedding Soup	Creamy Mustard Chicken with green beans
SUN	Acai Smoothie	Caesar Salad	Cashew Chicken Strips with Escarole Salad

WEEK 3 MEAL PLANS

DAY 1

BREAKFAST:

Cloud bread Separate 3 room temperature **eggs**. Place whites in a medium bowl and yolks in another bowl. Add 3 tbsp of **cream cheese** to egg whites and mix well. Add ¼ tsp **cream of tartar** and ¼ tsp **salt** to cream cheese mixture and mix at high speed with mixer until stiff peaks form. Slowly fold egg yolks into mixture until well combined. Preheat oven to 300° F and line two baking sheets with parchment paper. Divide batter into six equal portions and bake for 30 minutes. Cool and enjoy. *Double recipe for pizza crust for Day 2 lunch.*

LUNCH:

Cobb Salad: Romaine **lettuce** topped with **grilled chicken** or ham, diced **hardboiled eggs**, **bacon**, **cheese**, **avocado slices** and full fat ranch or blue cheese **dressing**.

DINNER:

Cauliflower Bacon Bake Preheat oven to 350° F. Microwave 1 large **cauliflower**, cut into small pieces, for 2 minutes. In a medium pot, melt 1 tbsp **butter**, 2 oz **cream cheese**, 1 cup **heavy cream**, and 1 cup shredded **cheddar cheese**, stirring until smooth. Add salt & pepper. In a glass baking dish, add the steamed cauliflower, cheese sauce and 5 slices of **bacon**, cooked and crumbled. Cover with 1/4 cup shredded cheddar cheese. Bake for 30 minutes or until cheese is melted.

SNACKS:

Salami and string cheese

½ cup macadamia nuts + 2 squares dark chocolate

WATER INTAKE:

WEEK 3 MEAL PLANS

DAY 2

BREAKFAST:

Eggs Benedict with hollandaise sauce Lightly grease skillet. Fill skillet half way with water and. Bring water to boiling. Reduce heat & simmer. Break 4 **eggs** into cup & carefully slide one at a time into water. Simmer for 5 minutes & remove. Remove poached egg & serve with warm **Canadian Bacon** & Hollandaise Sauce (combine 1/2 cup **butter**, 3 beaten **egg yolks**, 1 **tbsp water**, 1 tbsp **lemon juice** and heat in double boiler, stirring constantly).

LUNCH:

Cloud Bread Pizza

Mix 4 tbsp **tomato sauce** with ¼ tsp **garlic salt** and dash of **oregano**. Spread on **bread** (see Day 1 recipe) and add **toppings** such as pepperoni or sausage and **mozzarella cheese**. Bake at 375° F for 5-8 minutes or until cheese is melted.

DINNER:

Slow Swedish Meatballs with cabbage pasta

For sauce, mix 1 cup **beef broth** with 8 oz of **cream cheese**. For Meatballs, mix 1 lb **ground beef** with ¾ 1lb ground pork or **sausage** with 1 egg, ¼ cup **tomato sauce** and 2 tsp **salt**. Form into balls. Place meatballs in crock pot with sauce. Cover and cook on high for 2 hours or low for 4 hours. For "pasta," shred **cabbage** and sauté in coconut oil until tender, about 15 minutes.

SNACKS:

Apples with cream cheese

2 squares dark chocolate and pumpkin seeds

WATER INTAKE:

WEEK 3 MEAL PLANS

DAY 3

BREAKFAST:

Chia seed coconut pudding with raspberries Mix one 15 oz can full fat **coconut milk** with ½ cup **chia seeds**. Seal in airtight container and refrigerate 4 hours or overnight. Super easy just needs to be done ahead of time! Optional, add 1 tbsp nut butter.

LUNCH:

Salmon Cakes with Lemon Butter Sauce Mix one **egg** with ½ tsp **salt**, 1 tbsp **lemon juice**, and one 14.5 oz **can of wild salmon**, drained. Add 2-4 tbsp **coconut flour** until dry enough to form into patties. Heat up a large pan over medium heat. Add a 2-4 tbsp of butter or coconut oil. Once melted, cook salmon until golden brown, about 5 minutes per side. For sauce, mix together ½ up **butter** with 1 tsp **lemon zest** (or 1 tbsp lemon juice) with 2 tbsp of drained **caper**s. Serve with chopped **asparagu**s microwaved for 2 minutes. *Can be made night before and reheated.*

DINNER:

Ensenada chicken & Brussels Sprouts & Salad Marinate four **chicken breasts** in sealable plastic bag in 4 tbsp **olive oil**, 3 tbsp **chili powder**, 3 tsp **cumin**, 1 tsp **salt** for 30 minutes in fridge. Oil grill or skillet and cook on medium high heat for 3-5 minutes each side or until cooked. Serve with avocado, sour cream, and salsa. Quarter **Brussels Sprouts** and drizzle with 1 tbsp olive oil and ½ tsp kosher salt. Roast at 425° F for 20 minutes.

SNACKS:

Kale chips with sour cream Clean, remove stems, and pat **kale** leaves dry. Cut into bite size pieces and spray with olive oil. Roast for 350° F for 10-15 minutes. Works well with Brussels sprouts as well. Roast for 8-10 minutes.

Blueberries and almonds

WATER INTAKE:

WEEK 3 MEAL PLANS

DAY 4

BREAKFAST:

Scrambled eggs with sausage

LUNCH:

Fajita Bowl Leftover Ensenada **chicken** with sautéed **onion**s and **bell peppers** with chopped **avocado**, cilantro, **sour cream**, **salsa** and **cheese**. If you don't have leftover chicken, sauté chicken in equal parts soy sauce & white vinegar.

DINNER:

Gyoza Filling Wraps Mix 1 lb **ground pork,** one **egg**, 1 tbsp **soy sauce**, 1 tbsp **sesame oil** with ½ head **cabbage**, chopped finely. Sauté in olive oil as needed in heated pan until thoroughly cooked. Serve in romaine wraps with sliced red pepper and cilantro. drizzle with dipping sauce. Dipping sauce: mix 2 tbsp **balsamic vinegar**, 1 tbsp **sesame oil** and 1 tbsp **soy sauce** (add water if you want to thin it out).

SNACKS:

Bell Peppers & cucumber in guacamole

Deviled eggs

WATER INTAKE:

WEEK 3 MEAL PLANS

DAY 5

BREAKFAST:

Chocolate Peanut Butter Smoothie In blender, pulse together 1/4 cup **peanut butter** with 2 tbsp **cocoa powder** and ½ cup **heavy cream** (or coconut cream), protein powder (optional) and ¾ cup **almond milk.**

LUNCH:

Goat Cheese salad Preheat the oven to 400° F. Slice **goat cheese** and place in a greased baking dish and bake for 10 minutes. In a skillet, melt two tbsp of **butter** and add 1 tbsp **balsamic vinegar** and bring to a boil. Simmer for two minutes and remove from heat. Serve goat cheese with balsamic butter over **spinach** with toasted **pumpkin seeds**.

DINNER:

Greek Chicken Bake
Place sliced **zucchini, red bell pepper** and **onion** in a large casserole dish. Place four boneless **chicken breasts** on top. In a small bowl, mix together 1/3 cup olive oil, 1 tsp **oregano,** ½ tsp **rosemary,** ½ tsp **salt** and pour over chicken and veggies. Bake covered for 35 minutes at 375 ° F. Crumble **feta cheese** over the top and sprinkle with 3 tbsp of **balsamic vinegar** and serve.

SNACKS:

Cheese and pistachios

Greek yogurt and berries

WATER INTAKE:

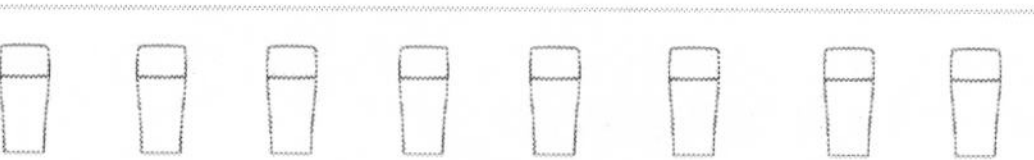

WEEK 3 MEAL PLANS

DAY 6

BREAKFAST:

Fried eggs with spinach sautéed in butter

LUNCH:

Italian Wedding Soup Heat 2 tbsp **olive oil** in a large saucepan over medium heat. Add a diced yellow **onion** and cook until tender. Stir in diced **garlic** and cook for another minute. Add six cups **chicken broth**, 1 tsp **oregano**, 1 tsp **thyme** and simmer for 10 minutes. Stir in 1 cup **cauliflower rice** and 10 small **meatball**s. Cook until heated. Stir in 2 cups fresh **spinach** and cook until wilted. Salt and pepper to taste and serve.

DINNER:

Creamy Mustard Chicken Toast 1 cup sliced **mushrooms** in a nonstick pan on medium-high heat for several minutes. Add sliced **red onion** and two **chicken breasts** that have been cut into strips and 3 tbsp of **olive oil**. Cook for 5 minutes, stirring often. Add 2 tsp whole-grain **mustard** and ¼ cup **heavy cream** and 2/3 cup of **water.** Bring to a boil, then reduce heat and simmer until chicken is cooked through and the sauce is a nice consistency. Salt, pepper & serve with steamed or microwaved green beans.

SNACKS:

Blueberries and whipped cream

Peanut Butter Fat Bomb Mix ¼ cup **cocoa powder** with ½ cup **peanut butter** and ¼ cup melted **coconut oil**. Stir until smooth and pour into ice cube trays and put in freezer until set. Store in airtight container in refrigerator.

WATER INTAKE:

WEEK 3 MEAL PLANS

DAY 7

BREAKFAST:

Acai Smoothie Blend together 1 packet unsweetened **Acai puree** (100 grams) with 1 tbsp plain **Greek Yogurt** and ¼ cup **coconut milk**, almond milk or heavy cream plus 2 drops of liquid **stevia** or to taste. Thin with water if necessary. Optional, blend in ½ avocado for more fat. *If you can't find acai, use frozen berries.*

LUNCH:

Caesar Salad **Romaine lettuce**, leftover pesto **chicken**, grated **parmesan cheese** with Caesar dressing (bottled or mix 4 tbsp **lemon juice** with ¼ cup **olive oil**, 1 /2 tsp **Worcestershire sauce**, ½ tsp salt, 1 clove of **garlic**, peeled & smashed, 1 raw **egg**, ½ cup **Parmesan cheese**, 1 tsp pepper, and squeeze of **anchovy paste**)

DINNER:

Cashew Chicken Strips with Salad Pulse ½ cup roasted cashews in a food processor with 1 tsp salt. Cut chicken breasts into strips and dip in beaten egg, then crushed cashews. Bake at 375 ° F for 25-35 minutes. **Escarole Salad:** Toss together a head of chopped **escarole** with 1/2 cup of grated **parmesan cheese** and pickled **red onions**. Drizzle with balsamic vinegar and olive oil. **Pickled onion:** Combine 1/2 cup **red wine vinegar** with 1/2 cup **water**. Stir in 1 tbsp **salt**. Add a **red onion**, sliced into rings and let sit for at least an hour to overnight.

SNACKS:

Almonds and string cheese

Peanut Butter Cookies: Mix together 1 **egg** with 1 tsp **vanill**a and 2 drops of liquid **stevia**. Stir in ¾ cup of **peanut butter** (or almond) and 2 tsp of **blanched almond** flour (optional). Roll into balls and put on cookie sheet lined with parchment paper or sprayed aluminum foil. Bake at 350° F for 12 minutes.

WATER INTAKE:

SELF-CARE IDEAS

TYPE	THINK ABOUT	IMPORTANT TO YOU
PHYSICAL	sleep daily exercise healthy food drink water rest	
SPIRITUAL	alone time meditation time in nature creating	
SOCIAL	set boundaries positive social media connection build relationships	
EMOTIONAL	forgive others and yourself have compassion be kind	

NOTES

SELF-CARE IDEAS

TYPE	THINK ABOUT	IMPORTANT TO YOU
PERSONAL	try new hobbies revisit old hobbies be true to yourself learn a language be vulnerable	
MONEY	save money spend wisely budget treat yourself	
HOME	organize your space healthy environment declutter	
CAREER	manage your time healthy boundaries take time to rest work/life balance know your worth	

NOTES

WEEK 1: SELF-CARE

DATE

FOCUS FOR THE WEEK:

SELF CARE CHECKLIST:

- [ ]
- [ ]
- [ ]
- [ ]
- [ ]
- [ ]
- [ ]
- [ ]
- [ ]
- [ ]

WHAT MOTIVATES ME:

SELF CARE CHECKLIST

GOALS	M	T	W	T	F	S	S
Got enough rest	○	○	○	○	○	○	○
Drank water	○	○	○	○	○	○	○
Exercised	○	○	○	○	○	○	○
Ate Mindfully	○	○	○	○	○	○	○
____________	○	○	○	○	○	○	○
____________	○	○	○	○	○	○	○
____________	○	○	○	○	○	○	○
____________	○	○	○	○	○	○	○
____________	○	○	○	○	○	○	○
____________	○	○	○	○	○	○	○
____________	○	○	○	○	○	○	○

WEEK 1: OVERVIEW

DAILY PLAN
MON:
TUES:
WED:
THUR:
FRI:
SAT:
SUN:

TO DO LIST:

NOTES & REMINDERS

THOUGHTS

WEEK 1: TOP 3 GOALS

GOAL	STEPS TO MAKE IT HAPPEN	DATE	✓

GOAL	STEPS TO MAKE IT HAPPEN	DATE	✓

GOAL	STEPS TO MAKE IT HAPPEN	DATE	✓

WEEK 1: EXERCISE

MON	
TUE	
WED	
THUR	
FRI	
SAT	
SUN	

INTERMITTENT FASTING *Tracker*

WEEK OF:

Monday

Goal	12	1	2	3	4	5	6	7	8	9	10	11	12	1	2	3	4	5	6	7	8	9	10	11
Actual	12	1	2	3	4	5	6	7	8	9	10	11	12	1	2	3	4	5	6	7	8	9	10	11

Tuesday

Goal	12	1	2	3	4	5	6	7	8	9	10	11	12	1	2	3	4	5	6	7	8	9	10	11
Actual	12	1	2	3	4	5	6	7	8	9	10	11	12	1	2	3	4	5	6	7	8	9	10	11

Wednesday

Goal	12	1	2	3	4	5	6	7	8	9	10	11	12	1	2	3	4	5	6	7	8	9	10	11
Actual	12	1	2	3	4	5	6	7	8	9	10	11	12	1	2	3	4	5	6	7	8	9	10	11

Thursday

Goal	12	1	2	3	4	5	6	7	8	9	10	11	12	1	2	3	4	5	6	7	8	9	10	11
Actual	12	1	2	3	4	5	6	7	8	9	10	11	12	1	2	3	4	5	6	7	8	9	10	11

Friday

Goal	12	1	2	3	4	5	6	7	8	9	10	11	12	1	2	3	4	5	6	7	8	9	10	11
Actual	12	1	2	3	4	5	6	7	8	9	10	11	12	1	2	3	4	5	6	7	8	9	10	11

Saturday

Goal	12	1	2	3	4	5	6	7	8	9	10	11	12	1	2	3	4	5	6	7	8	9	10	11
Actual	12	1	2	3	4	5	6	7	8	9	10	11	12	1	2	3	4	5	6	7	8	9	10	11

Sunday

Goal	12	1	2	3	4	5	6	7	8	9	10	11	12	1	2	3	4	5	6	7	8	9	10	11
Actual	12	1	2	3	4	5	6	7	8	9	10	11	12	1	2	3	4	5	6	7	8	9	10	11

WEEK 1: MEAL PLANS

	BREAKFAST	LUNCH	DINNER
MON			
TUES			
WED			
THU			
FRI			
SAT			
SUN			

SHOPPING LIST

WEEK 1: FOOD JOURNAL

Day 1

DATE:

BREAKFAST: carbs:

LUNCH: carbs:

DINNER: carbs:

SNACKS: carbs:

WATER INTAKE:

WEEK 1: FOOD JOURNAL

Day 2

DATE:

BREAKFAST: carbs:

LUNCH: carbs:

DINNER: carbs:

SNACKS: carbs:

WATER INTAKE:

WEEK 1: FOOD JOURNAL

Day 3

DATE:

BREAKFAST: *carbs:*

LUNCH: *carbs:*

DINNER: *carbs:*

SNACKS: *carbs:*

WATER INTAKE:

WEEK 1: FOOD JOURNAL

Day 4

DATE:

BREAKFAST: carbs:

LUNCH: carbs:

DINNER: carbs:

SNACKS: carbs:

WATER INTAKE:

WEEK 1: FOOD JOURNAL

Day 5

DATE:

BREAKFAST: carbs:

LUNCH: carbs:

DINNER: carbs:

SNACKS: carbs:

WATER INTAKE:

WEEK 1: FOOD JOURNAL

Day 6

DATE:

BREAKFAST: *carbs:*

LUNCH: *carbs:*

DINNER: *carbs:*

SNACKS: *carbs:*

WATER INTAKE:

WEEK 1: FOOD JOURNAL

Day 7

DATE:

BREAKFAST: *carbs:*

LUNCH: *carbs:*

DINNER: *carbs:*

SNACKS: *carbs:*

WATER INTAKE:

WEEK 1: RESULTS

DATE:

	MEASUREMENT:	LOSS/GAIN:
WEIGHT:		
LEFT ARM:		
RIGHT ARM:		
CHEST:		
WAIST:		
HIPS:		
LEFT THIGH:		
RIGHT THIGH:		

Weekly Goals

WEEK 2: SELF-CARE

DATE

SELF CARE CHECKLIST:

FOCUS FOR THE WEEK:

WHAT MOTIVATES ME:

SELF CARE CHECKLIST

GOALS	M	T	W	T	F	S	S
Got enough rest	○	○	○	○	○	○	○
Drank water	○	○	○	○	○	○	○
Exercised	○	○	○	○	○	○	○
Ate Mindfully	○	○	○	○	○	○	○
______________	○	○	○	○	○	○	○
______________	○	○	○	○	○	○	○
______________	○	○	○	○	○	○	○
______________	○	○	○	○	○	○	○
______________	○	○	○	○	○	○	○
______________	○	○	○	○	○	○	○
______________	○	○	○	○	○	○	○

WEEK 2: OVERVIEW

DAILY PLAN

MON:

TUES:

WED:

THUR:

FRI:

SAT:

SUN:

TO DO LIST:

NOTES & REMINDERS

THOUGHTS

WEEK 2: TOP 3 GOALS

GOAL	STEPS TO MAKE IT HAPPEN	DATE	✓

GOAL	STEPS TO MAKE IT HAPPEN	DATE	✓

GOAL	STEPS TO MAKE IT HAPPEN	DATE	✓

WEEK 2: EXERCISE

MON	
TUE	
WED	
THUR	
FRI	
SAT	
SUN	

INTERMITTENT FASTING *Tracker*

WEEK OF:

Monday

Goal	12	1	2	3	4	5	6	7	8	9	10	11	12	1	2	3	4	5	6	7	8	9	10	11
Actual	12	1	2	3	4	5	6	7	8	9	10	11	12	1	2	3	4	5	6	7	8	9	10	11

Tuesday

Goal	12	1	2	3	4	5	6	7	8	9	10	11	12	1	2	3	4	5	6	7	8	9	10	11
Actual	12	1	2	3	4	5	6	7	8	9	10	11	12	1	2	3	4	5	6	7	8	9	10	11

Wednesday

Goal	12	1	2	3	4	5	6	7	8	9	10	11	12	1	2	3	4	5	6	7	8	9	10	11
Actual	12	1	2	3	4	5	6	7	8	9	10	11	12	1	2	3	4	5	6	7	8	9	10	11

Thursday

Goal	12	1	2	3	4	5	6	7	8	9	10	11	12	1	2	3	4	5	6	7	8	9	10	11
Actual	12	1	2	3	4	5	6	7	8	9	10	11	12	1	2	3	4	5	6	7	8	9	10	11

Friday

Goal	12	1	2	3	4	5	6	7	8	9	10	11	12	1	2	3	4	5	6	7	8	9	10	11
Actual	12	1	2	3	4	5	6	7	8	9	10	11	12	1	2	3	4	5	6	7	8	9	10	11

Saturday

Goal	12	1	2	3	4	5	6	7	8	9	10	11	12	1	2	3	4	5	6	7	8	9	10	11
Actual	12	1	2	3	4	5	6	7	8	9	10	11	12	1	2	3	4	5	6	7	8	9	10	11

Sunday

Goal	12	1	2	3	4	5	6	7	8	9	10	11	12	1	2	3	4	5	6	7	8	9	10	11
Actual	12	1	2	3	4	5	6	7	8	9	10	11	12	1	2	3	4	5	6	7	8	9	10	11

WEEK 2: MEAL PLANS

	BREAKFAST	LUNCH	DINNER
MON			
TUES			
WED			
THU			
FRI			
SAT			
SUN			

SHOPPING LIST

WEEK 2: FOOD JOURNAL

Day 1

DATE:

BREAKFAST: *carbs:*

LUNCH: *carbs:*

DINNER: *carbs:*

SNACKS: *carbs:*

WATER INTAKE:

WEEK 2: FOOD JOURNAL

Day 2

DATE:

BREAKFAST: *carbs:*

LUNCH: *carbs:*

DINNER: *carbs:*

SNACKS: *carbs:*

WATER INTAKE:

WEEK 2: FOOD JOURNAL

Day 3

DATE:

BREAKFAST: *carbs:*

LUNCH: *carbs:*

DINNER: *carbs:*

SNACKS: *carbs:*

WATER INTAKE:

WEEK 2: FOOD JOURNAL

Day 4

DATE:

BREAKFAST: *carbs:*

LUNCH: *carbs:*

DINNER: *carbs:*

SNACKS: *carbs:*

WATER INTAKE:

WEEK 2: FOOD JOURNAL

Day 5

DATE:

BREAKFAST: *carbs:*

LUNCH: *carbs:*

DINNER: *carbs:*

SNACKS: *carbs:*

WATER INTAKE:

WEEK 2: FOOD JOURNAL

Day 6

DATE:

BREAKFAST: *carbs:*

LUNCH: *carbs:*

DINNER: *carbs:*

SNACKS: *carbs:*

WATER INTAKE:

WEEK 2: FOOD JOURNAL

Day 7

DATE:

BREAKFAST: *carbs:*

LUNCH: *carbs:*

DINNER: *carbs:*

SNACKS: *carbs:*

WATER INTAKE:

WEEK 2: RESULTS

DATE:

	MEASUREMENT:	LOSS/GAIN:
WEIGHT:		
LEFT ARM:		
RIGHT ARM:		
CHEST:		
WAIST:		
HIPS:		
LEFT THIGH:		
RIGHT THIGH:		

Weekly Goals

WEEK 3: SELF-CARE

DATE

SELF CARE CHECKLIST:

FOCUS FOR THE WEEK:

WHAT MOTIVATES ME:

SELF CARE CHECKLIST

GOALS	M	T	W	T	F	S	S
Got enough rest							
Drank water							
Exercised							
Ate Mindfully							
______							
______							
______							
______							
______							
______							
______							

WEEK 3: OVERVIEW

DAILY PLAN

MON:

TUES:

WED:

THUR:

FRI:

SAT:

SUN:

TO DO LIST:

NOTES & REMINDERS

THOUGHTS

WEEK 3: TOP 3 GOALS

GOAL	STEPS TO MAKE IT HAPPEN	DATE	✓

GOAL	STEPS TO MAKE IT HAPPEN	DATE	✓

GOAL	STEPS TO MAKE IT HAPPEN	DATE	✓

WEEK 3: EXERCISE

MON	
TUE	
WED	
THUR	
FRI	
SAT	
SUN	

INTERMITTENT FASTING *Tracker*

WEEK OF:

Monday

Goal	12	1	2	3	4	5	6	7	8	9	10	11	12	1	2	3	4	5	6	7	8	9	10	11
Actual	12	1	2	3	4	5	6	7	8	9	10	11	12	1	2	3	4	5	6	7	8	9	10	11

Tuesday

Goal	12	1	2	3	4	5	6	7	8	9	10	11	12	1	2	3	4	5	6	7	8	9	10	11
Actual	12	1	2	3	4	5	6	7	8	9	10	11	12	1	2	3	4	5	6	7	8	9	10	11

Wednesday

Goal	12	1	2	3	4	5	6	7	8	9	10	11	12	1	2	3	4	5	6	7	8	9	10	11
Actual	12	1	2	3	4	5	6	7	8	9	10	11	12	1	2	3	4	5	6	7	8	9	10	11

Thursday

Goal	12	1	2	3	4	5	6	7	8	9	10	11	12	1	2	3	4	5	6	7	8	9	10	11
Actual	12	1	2	3	4	5	6	7	8	9	10	11	12	1	2	3	4	5	6	7	8	9	10	11

Friday

Goal	12	1	2	3	4	5	6	7	8	9	10	11	12	1	2	3	4	5	6	7	8	9	10	11
Actual	12	1	2	3	4	5	6	7	8	9	10	11	12	1	2	3	4	5	6	7	8	9	10	11

Saturday

Goal	12	1	2	3	4	5	6	7	8	9	10	11	12	1	2	3	4	5	6	7	8	9	10	11
Actual	12	1	2	3	4	5	6	7	8	9	10	11	12	1	2	3	4	5	6	7	8	9	10	11

Sunday

Goal	12	1	2	3	4	5	6	7	8	9	10	11	12	1	2	3	4	5	6	7	8	9	10	11
Actual	12	1	2	3	4	5	6	7	8	9	10	11	12	1	2	3	4	5	6	7	8	9	10	11

WEEK 3: MEAL PLANS

	BREAKFAST	LUNCH	DINNER
MON			
TUES			
WED			
THU			
FRI			
SAT			
SUN			

SHOPPING LIST

WEEK 3: FOOD JOURNAL

Day 1

DATE:

BREAKFAST: *carbs:*

LUNCH: *carbs:*

DINNER: *carbs:*

SNACKS: *carbs:*

WATER INTAKE:

WEEK 3: FOOD JOURNAL

Day 2

DATE:

BREAKFAST: *carbs:*

LUNCH: *carbs:*

DINNER: *carbs:*

SNACKS: *carbs:*

WATER INTAKE:

WEEK 3: FOOD JOURNAL

Day 3

DATE:

BREAKFAST: carbs:

LUNCH: carbs:

DINNER: carbs:

SNACKS: carbs:

WATER INTAKE:

WEEK 3: FOOD JOURNAL

Day 4

DATE:

BREAKFAST: carbs:

LUNCH: carbs:

DINNER: carbs:

SNACKS: carbs:

WATER INTAKE:

WEEK 3: FOOD JOURNAL

Day 5

DATE:

BREAKFAST: carbs:

LUNCH: carbs:

DINNER: carbs:

SNACKS: carbs:

WATER INTAKE:

WEEK 3: FOOD JOURNAL

Day 6

DATE:

BREAKFAST: carbs:

LUNCH: carbs:

DINNER: carbs:

SNACKS: carbs:

WATER INTAKE:

WEEK 3: FOOD JOURNAL

Day 7

DATE:

BREAKFAST: *carbs:*

LUNCH: *carbs:*

DINNER: *carbs:*

SNACKS: *carbs:*

WATER INTAKE:

WEEK 3: RESULTS

DATE:

	MEASUREMENT:	LOSS/GAIN:
WEIGHT:		
LEFT ARM:		
RIGHT ARM:		
CHEST:		
WAIST:		
HIPS:		
LEFT THIGH:		
RIGHT THIGH:		

Weekly Goals

WEEK 4: SELF-CARE

DATE

SELF CARE CHECKLIST:

FOCUS FOR THE WEEK:

WHAT MOTIVATES ME:

SELF CARE CHECKLIST

GOALS	M	T	W	T	F	S	S
Got enough rest	○	○	○	○	○	○	○
Drank water	○	○	○	○	○	○	○
Exercised	○	○	○	○	○	○	○
Ate Mindfully	○	○	○	○	○	○	○
____________	○	○	○	○	○	○	○
____________	○	○	○	○	○	○	○
____________	○	○	○	○	○	○	○
____________	○	○	○	○	○	○	○
____________	○	○	○	○	○	○	○
____________	○	○	○	○	○	○	○
____________	○	○	○	○	○	○	○

WEEK 4: OVERVIEW

DAILY PLAN
MON:
TUES:
WED:
THUR:
FRI:
SAT:
SUN:

TO DO LIST:

NOTES & REMINDERS

THOUGHTS

WEEK 4: TOP 3 GOALS

GOAL	STEPS TO MAKE IT HAPPEN	DATE	✓

GOAL	STEPS TO MAKE IT HAPPEN	DATE	✓

GOAL	STEPS TO MAKE IT HAPPEN	DATE	✓

WEEK 4: EXERCISE

MON	
TUE	
WED	
THUR	
FRI	
SAT	
SUN	

INTERMITTENT FASTING *Tracker*

WEEK OF:

Monday

Goal	12	1	2	3	4	5	6	7	8	9	10	11	12	1	2	3	4	5	6	7	8	9	10	11
Actual	12	1	2	3	4	5	6	7	8	9	10	11	12	1	2	3	4	5	6	7	8	9	10	11

Tuesday

Goal	12	1	2	3	4	5	6	7	8	9	10	11	12	1	2	3	4	5	6	7	8	9	10	11
Actual	12	1	2	3	4	5	6	7	8	9	10	11	12	1	2	3	4	5	6	7	8	9	10	11

Wednesday

Goal	12	1	2	3	4	5	6	7	8	9	10	11	12	1	2	3	4	5	6	7	8	9	10	11
Actual	12	1	2	3	4	5	6	7	8	9	10	11	12	1	2	3	4	5	6	7	8	9	10	11

Thursday

Goal	12	1	2	3	4	5	6	7	8	9	10	11	12	1	2	3	4	5	6	7	8	9	10	11
Actual	12	1	2	3	4	5	6	7	8	9	10	11	12	1	2	3	4	5	6	7	8	9	10	11

Friday

Goal	12	1	2	3	4	5	6	7	8	9	10	11	12	1	2	3	4	5	6	7	8	9	10	11
Actual	12	1	2	3	4	5	6	7	8	9	10	11	12	1	2	3	4	5	6	7	8	9	10	11

Saturday

Goal	12	1	2	3	4	5	6	7	8	9	10	11	12	1	2	3	4	5	6	7	8	9	10	11
Actual	12	1	2	3	4	5	6	7	8	9	10	11	12	1	2	3	4	5	6	7	8	9	10	11

Sunday

Goal	12	1	2	3	4	5	6	7	8	9	10	11	12	1	2	3	4	5	6	7	8	9	10	11
Actual	12	1	2	3	4	5	6	7	8	9	10	11	12	1	2	3	4	5	6	7	8	9	10	11

WEEK 4: MEAL PLANS

	BREAKFAST	LUNCH	DINNER
MON			
TUES			
WED			
THU			
FRI			
SAT			
SUN			

SHOPPING LIST

WEEK 4: FOOD JOURNAL

Day 1

DATE:

BREAKFAST: *carbs:*

LUNCH: *carbs:*

DINNER: *carbs:*

SNACKS: *carbs:*

WATER INTAKE:

WEEK 4: FOOD JOURNAL

Day 2

DATE:

BREAKFAST: *carbs:*

LUNCH: *carbs:*

DINNER: *carbs:*

SNACKS: *carbs:*

WATER INTAKE:

WEEK 4: FOOD JOURNAL

Day 3

DATE:

BREAKFAST: carbs:

LUNCH: carbs:

DINNER: carbs:

SNACKS: carbs:

WATER INTAKE:

WEEK 4: FOOD JOURNAL

Day 4

DATE:

BREAKFAST: carbs:

LUNCH: carbs:

DINNER: carbs:

SNACKS: carbs:

WATER INTAKE:

WEEK 4: FOOD JOURNAL

Day 5

DATE:

BREAKFAST: *carbs:*

LUNCH: *carbs:*

DINNER: *carbs:*

SNACKS: *carbs:*

WATER INTAKE:

WEEK 4: FOOD JOURNAL

Day 6

DATE:

BREAKFAST: *carbs:*

LUNCH: *carbs:*

DINNER: *carbs:*

SNACKS: *carbs:*

WATER INTAKE:

WEEK 4: FOOD JOURNAL

Day 7

DATE:

BREAKFAST: *carbs:*

LUNCH: *carbs:*

DINNER: *carbs:*

SNACKS: *carbs:*

WATER INTAKE:

WEEK 4: RESULTS

DATE:

	MEASUREMENT:	LOSS/GAIN:
WEIGHT:		
LEFT ARM:		
RIGHT ARM:		
CHEST:		
WAIST:		
HIPS:		
LEFT THIGH:		
RIGHT THIGH:		

Weekly Goals

WEEK 5: SELF-CARE

DATE

SELF CARE CHECKLIST:

FOCUS FOR THE WEEK:

WHAT MOTIVATES ME:

SELF CARE CHECKLIST

GOALS	M	T	W	T	F	S	S
Got enough rest	○	○	○	○	○	○	○
Drank water	○	○	○	○	○	○	○
Exercised	○	○	○	○	○	○	○
Ate Mindfully	○	○	○	○	○	○	○
________	○	○	○	○	○	○	○
________	○	○	○	○	○	○	○
________	○	○	○	○	○	○	○
________	○	○	○	○	○	○	○
________	○	○	○	○	○	○	○
________	○	○	○	○	○	○	○
________	○	○	○	○	○	○	○

WEEK 5: OVERVIEW

DAILY PLAN
MON:
TUES:
WED:
THUR:
FRI:
SAT:
SUN:

TO DO LIST:

- [ ]
- [ ]
- [ ]
- [ ]
- [ ]
- [ ]
- [ ]
- [ ]
- [ ]
- [ ]

NOTES & REMINDERS

THOUGHTS

WEEK 5: TOP 3 GOALS

GOAL	STEPS TO MAKE IT HAPPEN	DATE	✓

GOAL	STEPS TO MAKE IT HAPPEN	DATE	✓

GOAL	STEPS TO MAKE IT HAPPEN	DATE	✓

WEEK 5: EXERCISE

MON	
TUE	
WED	
THUR	
FRI	
SAT	
SUN	

INTERMITTENT FASTING
Tracker

WEEK OF:

Monday

Goal	12	1	2	3	4	5	6	7	8	9	10	11	12	1	2	3	4	5	6	7	8	9	10	11
Actual	12	1	2	3	4	5	6	7	8	9	10	11	12	1	2	3	4	5	6	7	8	9	10	11

Tuesday

Goal	12	1	2	3	4	5	6	7	8	9	10	11	12	1	2	3	4	5	6	7	8	9	10	11
Actual	12	1	2	3	4	5	6	7	8	9	10	11	12	1	2	3	4	5	6	7	8	9	10	11

Wednesday

Goal	12	1	2	3	4	5	6	7	8	9	10	11	12	1	2	3	4	5	6	7	8	9	10	11
Actual	12	1	2	3	4	5	6	7	8	9	10	11	12	1	2	3	4	5	6	7	8	9	10	11

Thursday

Goal	12	1	2	3	4	5	6	7	8	9	10	11	12	1	2	3	4	5	6	7	8	9	10	11
Actual	12	1	2	3	4	5	6	7	8	9	10	11	12	1	2	3	4	5	6	7	8	9	10	11

Friday

Goal	12	1	2	3	4	5	6	7	8	9	10	11	12	1	2	3	4	5	6	7	8	9	10	11
Actual	12	1	2	3	4	5	6	7	8	9	10	11	12	1	2	3	4	5	6	7	8	9	10	11

Saturday

Goal	12	1	2	3	4	5	6	7	8	9	10	11	12	1	2	3	4	5	6	7	8	9	10	11
Actual	12	1	2	3	4	5	6	7	8	9	10	11	12	1	2	3	4	5	6	7	8	9	10	11

Sunday

Goal	12	1	2	3	4	5	6	7	8	9	10	11	12	1	2	3	4	5	6	7	8	9	10	11
Actual	12	1	2	3	4	5	6	7	8	9	10	11	12	1	2	3	4	5	6	7	8	9	10	11

WEEK 5: MEAL PLANS

	BREAKFAST	LUNCH	DINNER
MON			
TUES			
WED			
THU			
FRI			
SAT			
SUN			

SHOPPING LIST

WEEK 5: FOOD JOURNAL

Day 1

DATE:

BREAKFAST: *carbs:*

LUNCH: *carbs:*

DINNER: *carbs:*

SNACKS: *carbs:*

WATER INTAKE:

WEEK 5: FOOD JOURNAL

Day 2

DATE:

BREAKFAST: *carbs:*

LUNCH: *carbs:*

DINNER: *carbs:*

SNACKS: *carbs:*

WATER INTAKE:

WEEK 5: FOOD JOURNAL

Day 3

DATE:

BREAKFAST: carbs:

LUNCH: carbs:

DINNER: carbs:

SNACKS: carbs:

WATER INTAKE:

WEEK 5: FOOD JOURNAL

Day 4

DATE:

BREAKFAST: *carbs:*

LUNCH: *carbs:*

DINNER: *carbs:*

SNACKS: *carbs:*

WATER INTAKE:

WEEK 5: FOOD JOURNAL

Day 5

DATE:

BREAKFAST: carbs:

LUNCH: carbs:

DINNER: carbs:

SNACKS: carbs:

WATER INTAKE:

WEEK 5: FOOD JOURNAL

Day 6

DATE:

BREAKFAST: *carbs:*

LUNCH: *carbs:*

DINNER: *carbs:*

SNACKS: *carbs:*

WATER INTAKE:

WEEK 5: FOOD JOURNAL

Day 7

DATE:

BREAKFAST: carbs:

LUNCH: carbs:

DINNER: carbs:

SNACKS: carbs:

WATER INTAKE:

WEEK 5: RESULTS

DATE:

	MEASUREMENT:	LOSS/GAIN:
WEIGHT:		
LEFT ARM:		
RIGHT ARM:		
CHEST:		
WAIST:		
HIPS:		
LEFT THIGH:		
RIGHT THIGH:		

Weekly Goals

WEEK 6: SELF-CARE

DATE

SELF CARE CHECKLIST:

FOCUS FOR THE WEEK:

WHAT MOTIVATES ME:

SELF CARE CHECKLIST

GOALS	M	T	W	T	F	S	S
Got enough rest	○	○	○	○	○	○	○
Drank water	○	○	○	○	○	○	○
Exercised	○	○	○	○	○	○	○
Ate Mindfully	○	○	○	○	○	○	○
____________	○	○	○	○	○	○	○
____________	○	○	○	○	○	○	○
____________	○	○	○	○	○	○	○
____________	○	○	○	○	○	○	○
____________	○	○	○	○	○	○	○
____________	○	○	○	○	○	○	○
____________	○	○	○	○	○	○	○

WEEK 6: OVERVIEW

DAILY PLAN
MON:
TUES:
WED:
THUR:
FRI:
SAT:
SUN:

TO DO LIST:

NOTES & REMINDERS

THOUGHTS

WEEK 6: TOP 3 GOALS

GOAL	STEPS TO MAKE IT HAPPEN	DATE	✓

GOAL	STEPS TO MAKE IT HAPPEN	DATE	✓

GOAL	STEPS TO MAKE IT HAPPEN	DATE	✓

WEEK 6: EXERCISE

MON	
TUE	
WED	
THUR	
FRI	
SAT	
SUN	

INTERMITTENT FASTING *Tracker*

WEEK OF:

Monday

Goal	12	1	2	3	4	5	6	7	8	9	10	11	12	1	2	3	4	5	6	7	8	9	10	11
Actual	12	1	2	3	4	5	6	7	8	9	10	11	12	1	2	3	4	5	6	7	8	9	10	11

Tuesday

Goal	12	1	2	3	4	5	6	7	8	9	10	11	12	1	2	3	4	5	6	7	8	9	10	11
Actual	12	1	2	3	4	5	6	7	8	9	10	11	12	1	2	3	4	5	6	7	8	9	10	11

Wednesday

Goal	12	1	2	3	4	5	6	7	8	9	10	11	12	1	2	3	4	5	6	7	8	9	10	11
Actual	12	1	2	3	4	5	6	7	8	9	10	11	12	1	2	3	4	5	6	7	8	9	10	11

Thursday

Goal	12	1	2	3	4	5	6	7	8	9	10	11	12	1	2	3	4	5	6	7	8	9	10	11
Actual	12	1	2	3	4	5	6	7	8	9	10	11	12	1	2	3	4	5	6	7	8	9	10	11

Friday

Goal	12	1	2	3	4	5	6	7	8	9	10	11	12	1	2	3	4	5	6	7	8	9	10	11
Actual	12	1	2	3	4	5	6	7	8	9	10	11	12	1	2	3	4	5	6	7	8	9	10	11

Saturday

Goal	12	1	2	3	4	5	6	7	8	9	10	11	12	1	2	3	4	5	6	7	8	9	10	11
Actual	12	1	2	3	4	5	6	7	8	9	10	11	12	1	2	3	4	5	6	7	8	9	10	11

Sunday

Goal	12	1	2	3	4	5	6	7	8	9	10	11	12	1	2	3	4	5	6	7	8	9	10	11
Actual	12	1	2	3	4	5	6	7	8	9	10	11	12	1	2	3	4	5	6	7	8	9	10	11

WEEK 6: MEAL PLANS

	BREAKFAST	LUNCH	DINNER
MON			
TUES			
WED			
THU			
FRI			
SAT			
SUN			

SHOPPING LIST

WEEK 6: FOOD JOURNAL

Day 1

DATE:

BREAKFAST: carbs:

LUNCH: carbs:

DINNER: carbs:

SNACKS: carbs:

WATER INTAKE:

WEEK 6: FOOD JOURNAL

Day 2

DATE:

BREAKFAST: *carbs:*

LUNCH: *carbs:*

DINNER: *carbs:*

SNACKS: *carbs:*

WATER INTAKE:

WEEK 6: FOOD JOURNAL

Day 3

DATE:

BREAKFAST: *carbs:*

LUNCH: *carbs:*

DINNER: *carbs:*

SNACKS: *carbs:*

WATER INTAKE:

WEEK 6: FOOD JOURNAL

Day 4

DATE:

BREAKFAST: carbs:

LUNCH: carbs:

DINNER: carbs:

SNACKS: carbs:

WATER INTAKE:

WEEK 6: FOOD JOURNAL

Day 5

DATE:

BREAKFAST: carbs:

LUNCH: carbs:

DINNER: carbs:

SNACKS: carbs:

WATER INTAKE:

WEEK 6: FOOD JOURNAL

Day 6

DATE:

BREAKFAST: *carbs:*

LUNCH: *carbs:*

DINNER: *carbs:*

SNACKS: *carbs:*

WATER INTAKE:

WEEK 6: FOOD JOURNAL

Day 7

DATE:

BREAKFAST: *carbs:*

LUNCH: *carbs:*

DINNER: *carbs:*

SNACKS: *carbs:*

WATER INTAKE:

WEEK 6: RESULTS

DATE:

	MEASUREMENT:	LOSS/GAIN:
WEIGHT:		
LEFT ARM:		
RIGHT ARM:		
CHEST:		
WAIST:		
HIPS:		
LEFT THIGH:		
RIGHT THIGH:		

Weekly Goals

WEEK 7: SELF-CARE

DATE

SELF CARE CHECKLIST:

FOCUS FOR THE WEEK:

WHAT MOTIVATES ME:

SELF CARE CHECKLIST

GOALS	M	T	W	T	F	S	S
Got enough rest	○	○	○	○	○	○	○
Drank water	○	○	○	○	○	○	○
Exercised	○	○	○	○	○	○	○
Ate Mindfully	○	○	○	○	○	○	○
________________	○	○	○	○	○	○	○
________________	○	○	○	○	○	○	○
________________	○	○	○	○	○	○	○
________________	○	○	○	○	○	○	○
________________	○	○	○	○	○	○	○
________________	○	○	○	○	○	○	○
________________	○	○	○	○	○	○	○

WEEK 7: OVERVIEW

DAILY PLAN

MON:

TUES:

WED:

THUR:

FRI:

SAT:

SUN:

TO DO LIST:

NOTES & REMINDERS

THOUGHTS

WEEK 7: TOP 3 GOALS

GOAL	STEPS TO MAKE IT HAPPEN	DATE	✓

GOAL	STEPS TO MAKE IT HAPPEN	DATE	✓

GOAL	STEPS TO MAKE IT HAPPEN	DATE	✓

WEEK 7: EXERCISE

MON	
TUE	
WED	
THUR	
FRI	
SAT	
SUN	

INTERMITTENT FASTING *Tracker*

WEEK OF:

Monday

Goal	12	1	2	3	4	5	6	7	8	9	10	11	12	1	2	3	4	5	6	7	8	9	10	11
Actual	12	1	2	3	4	5	6	7	8	9	10	11	12	1	2	3	4	5	6	7	8	9	10	11

Tuesday

Goal	12	1	2	3	4	5	6	7	8	9	10	11	12	1	2	3	4	5	6	7	8	9	10	11
Actual	12	1	2	3	4	5	6	7	8	9	10	11	12	1	2	3	4	5	6	7	8	9	10	11

Wednesday

Goal	12	1	2	3	4	5	6	7	8	9	10	11	12	1	2	3	4	5	6	7	8	9	10	11
Actual	12	1	2	3	4	5	6	7	8	9	10	11	12	1	2	3	4	5	6	7	8	9	10	11

Thursday

Goal	12	1	2	3	4	5	6	7	8	9	10	11	12	1	2	3	4	5	6	7	8	9	10	11
Actual	12	1	2	3	4	5	6	7	8	9	10	11	12	1	2	3	4	5	6	7	8	9	10	11

Friday

Goal	12	1	2	3	4	5	6	7	8	9	10	11	12	1	2	3	4	5	6	7	8	9	10	11
Actual	12	1	2	3	4	5	6	7	8	9	10	11	12	1	2	3	4	5	6	7	8	9	10	11

Saturday

Goal	12	1	2	3	4	5	6	7	8	9	10	11	12	1	2	3	4	5	6	7	8	9	10	11
Actual	12	1	2	3	4	5	6	7	8	9	10	11	12	1	2	3	4	5	6	7	8	9	10	11

Sunday

Goal	12	1	2	3	4	5	6	7	8	9	10	11	12	1	2	3	4	5	6	7	8	9	10	11
Actual	12	1	2	3	4	5	6	7	8	9	10	11	12	1	2	3	4	5	6	7	8	9	10	11

WEEK 7: MEAL PLANS

	BREAKFAST	LUNCH	DINNER
MON			
TUES			
WED			
THU			
FRI			
SAT			
SUN			

SHOPPING LIST

WEEK 7: FOOD JOURNAL

Day 1

DATE:

BREAKFAST: carbs:

LUNCH: carbs:

DINNER: carbs:

SNACKS: carbs:

WATER INTAKE:

WEEK 7: FOOD JOURNAL

Day 2

DATE:

BREAKFAST: *carbs:*

LUNCH: *carbs:*

DINNER: *carbs:*

SNACKS: *carbs:*

WATER INTAKE:

WEEK 7: FOOD JOURNAL

Day 3

DATE:

BREAKFAST: *carbs:*

LUNCH: *carbs:*

DINNER: *carbs:*

SNACKS: *carbs:*

WATER INTAKE:

WEEK 7: FOOD JOURNAL

Day 4

DATE:

BREAKFAST: *carbs:*

LUNCH: *carbs:*

DINNER: *carbs:*

SNACKS: *carbs:*

WATER INTAKE:

WEEK 7: FOOD JOURNAL

Day 5

DATE:

BREAKFAST: *carbs:*

LUNCH: *carbs:*

DINNER: *carbs:*

SNACKS: *carbs:*

WATER INTAKE:

WEEK 7: FOOD JOURNAL

Day 6

DATE:

BREAKFAST: *carbs:*

LUNCH: *carbs:*

DINNER: *carbs:*

SNACKS: *carbs:*

WATER INTAKE:

WEEK 7: FOOD JOURNAL

Day 7

DATE:

BREAKFAST: carbs:

LUNCH: carbs:

DINNER: carbs:

SNACKS: carbs:

WATER INTAKE:

WEEK 7: RESULTS

DATE:

	MEASUREMENT:	LOSS/GAIN:
WEIGHT:		
LEFT ARM:		
RIGHT ARM:		
CHEST:		
WAIST:		
HIPS:		
LEFT THIGH:		
RIGHT THIGH:		

Weekly Goals

WEEK 8: SELF-CARE

DATE

SELF CARE CHECKLIST:

FOCUS FOR THE WEEK:

WHAT MOTIVATES ME:

SELF CARE CHECKLIST

GOALS	M	T	W	T	F	S	S
Got enough rest	○	○	○	○	○	○	○
Drank water	○	○	○	○	○	○	○
Exercised	○	○	○	○	○	○	○
Ate Mindfully	○	○	○	○	○	○	○
________________	○	○	○	○	○	○	○
________________	○	○	○	○	○	○	○
________________	○	○	○	○	○	○	○
________________	○	○	○	○	○	○	○
________________	○	○	○	○	○	○	○
________________	○	○	○	○	○	○	○
________________	○	○	○	○	○	○	○

WEEK 8: OVERVIEW

DAILY PLAN

MON:

TUES:

WED:

THUR:

FRI:

SAT:

SUN:

TO DO LIST:

NOTES & REMINDERS

THOUGHTS

WEEK 8: TOP 3 GOALS

GOAL	STEPS TO MAKE IT HAPPEN	DATE	✓

GOAL	STEPS TO MAKE IT HAPPEN	DATE	✓

GOAL	STEPS TO MAKE IT HAPPEN	DATE	✓

WEEK 8: EXERCISE

MON	
TUE	
WED	
THUR	
FRI	
SAT	
SUN	

INTERMITTENT FASTING *Tracker*

WEEK OF:

Monday																							
Goal	12	1	2	3	4	5	6	7	8	9	10	11	12	1	2	3	4	5	6	7	8	9	10	11
Actual	12	1	2	3	4	5	6	7	8	9	10	11	12	1	2	3	4	5	6	7	8	9	10	11

Tuesday																								
Goal	12	1	2	3	4	5	6	7	8	9	10	11	12	1	2	3	4	5	6	7	8	9	10	11
Actual	12	1	2	3	4	5	6	7	8	9	10	11	12	1	2	3	4	5	6	7	8	9	10	11

Wednesday																								
Goal	12	1	2	3	4	5	6	7	8	9	10	11	12	1	2	3	4	5	6	7	8	9	10	11
Actual	12	1	2	3	4	5	6	7	8	9	10	11	12	1	2	3	4	5	6	7	8	9	10	11

Thursday																								
Goal	12	1	2	3	4	5	6	7	8	9	10	11	12	1	2	3	4	5	6	7	8	9	10	11
Actual	12	1	2	3	4	5	6	7	8	9	10	11	12	1	2	3	4	5	6	7	8	9	10	11

Friday																								
Goal	12	1	2	3	4	5	6	7	8	9	10	11	12	1	2	3	4	5	6	7	8	9	10	11
Actual	12	1	2	3	4	5	6	7	8	9	10	11	12	1	2	3	4	5	6	7	8	9	10	11

Saturday																								
Goal	12	1	2	3	4	5	6	7	8	9	10	11	12	1	2	3	4	5	6	7	8	9	10	11
Actual	12	1	2	3	4	5	6	7	8	9	10	11	12	1	2	3	4	5	6	7	8	9	10	11

Sunday																								
Goal	12	1	2	3	4	5	6	7	8	9	10	11	12	1	2	3	4	5	6	7	8	9	10	11
Actual	12	1	2	3	4	5	6	7	8	9	10	11	12	1	2	3	4	5	6	7	8	9	10	11

WEEK 8: MEAL PLANS

	BREAKFAST	LUNCH	DINNER
MON			
TUES			
WED			
THU			
FRI			
SAT			
SUN			

SHOPPING LIST

WEEK 8: FOOD JOURNAL

Day 1

DATE:

BREAKFAST: carbs:

LUNCH: carbs:

DINNER: carbs:

SNACKS: carbs:

WATER INTAKE:

WEEK 8: FOOD JOURNAL

Day 2

DATE:

BREAKFAST: *carbs:*

LUNCH: *carbs:*

DINNER: *carbs:*

SNACKS: *carbs:*

WATER INTAKE:

WEEK 8: FOOD JOURNAL

Day 3

DATE:

BREAKFAST: carbs:

LUNCH: carbs:

DINNER: carbs:

SNACKS: carbs:

WATER INTAKE:

WEEK 8: FOOD JOURNAL

Day 4

DATE:

BREAKFAST: carbs:

LUNCH: carbs:

DINNER: carbs:

SNACKS: carbs:

WATER INTAKE:

WEEK 8: FOOD JOURNAL

Day 5

DATE:

BREAKFAST: carbs:

LUNCH: carbs:

DINNER: carbs:

SNACKS: carbs:

WATER INTAKE:

WEEK 8: FOOD JOURNAL

Day 6

DATE:

BREAKFAST: *carbs:*

LUNCH: *carbs:*

DINNER: *carbs:*

SNACKS: *carbs:*

WATER INTAKE:

WEEK 8: FOOD JOURNAL

Day 7

DATE:

BREAKFAST: carbs:

LUNCH: carbs:

DINNER: carbs:

SNACKS: carbs:

WATER INTAKE:

WEEK 8: RESULTS

DATE:

	MEASUREMENT:	LOSS/GAIN:
WEIGHT:		
LEFT ARM:		
RIGHT ARM:		
CHEST:		
WAIST:		
HIPS:		
LEFT THIGH:		
RIGHT THIGH:		

Weekly Goals

WEEK 9: SELF-CARE

DATE

SELF CARE CHECKLIST:

- [ ]
- [ ]
- [ ]
- [ ]
- [ ]
- [ ]
- [ ]
- [ ]
- [ ]
- [ ]

FOCUS FOR THE WEEK:

WHAT MOTIVATES ME:

SELF CARE CHECKLIST

GOALS	M	T	W	T	F	S	S
Got enough rest	○	○	○	○	○	○	○
Drank water	○	○	○	○	○	○	○
Exercised	○	○	○	○	○	○	○
Ate Mindfully	○	○	○	○	○	○	○
______________	○	○	○	○	○	○	○
______________	○	○	○	○	○	○	○
______________	○	○	○	○	○	○	○
______________	○	○	○	○	○	○	○
______________	○	○	○	○	○	○	○
______________	○	○	○	○	○	○	○
______________	○	○	○	○	○	○	○

WEEK 9: OVERVIEW

DAILY PLAN
MON:
TUES:
WED:
THUR:
FRI:
SAT:
SUN:

TO DO LIST:

NOTES & REMINDERS

THOUGHTS

WEEK 9: TOP 3 GOALS

GOAL	STEPS TO MAKE IT HAPPEN	DATE	✓

GOAL	STEPS TO MAKE IT HAPPEN	DATE	✓

GOAL	STEPS TO MAKE IT HAPPEN	DATE	✓

WEEK 9: EXERCISE

MON	
TUE	
WED	
THUR	
FRI	
SAT	
SUN	

INTERMITTENT FASTING *Tracker*

WEEK OF:

Monday

Goal	12	1	2	3	4	5	6	7	8	9	10	11	12	1	2	3	4	5	6	7	8	9	10	11
Actual	12	1	2	3	4	5	6	7	8	9	10	11	12	1	2	3	4	5	6	7	8	9	10	11

Tuesday

Goal	12	1	2	3	4	5	6	7	8	9	10	11	12	1	2	3	4	5	6	7	8	9	10	11
Actual	12	1	2	3	4	5	6	7	8	9	10	11	12	1	2	3	4	5	6	7	8	9	10	11

Wednesday

Goal	12	1	2	3	4	5	6	7	8	9	10	11	12	1	2	3	4	5	6	7	8	9	10	11
Actual	12	1	2	3	4	5	6	7	8	9	10	11	12	1	2	3	4	5	6	7	8	9	10	11

Thursday

Goal	12	1	2	3	4	5	6	7	8	9	10	11	12	1	2	3	4	5	6	7	8	9	10	11
Actual	12	1	2	3	4	5	6	7	8	9	10	11	12	1	2	3	4	5	6	7	8	9	10	11

Friday

Goal	12	1	2	3	4	5	6	7	8	9	10	11	12	1	2	3	4	5	6	7	8	9	10	11
Actual	12	1	2	3	4	5	6	7	8	9	10	11	12	1	2	3	4	5	6	7	8	9	10	11

Saturday

Goal	12	1	2	3	4	5	6	7	8	9	10	11	12	1	2	3	4	5	6	7	8	9	10	11
Actual	12	1	2	3	4	5	6	7	8	9	10	11	12	1	2	3	4	5	6	7	8	9	10	11

Sunday

Goal	12	1	2	3	4	5	6	7	8	9	10	11	12	1	2	3	4	5	6	7	8	9	10	11
Actual	12	1	2	3	4	5	6	7	8	9	10	11	12	1	2	3	4	5	6	7	8	9	10	11

WEEK 9: MEAL PLANS

	BREAKFAST	LUNCH	DINNER
MON			
TUES			
WED			
THU			
FRI			
SAT			
SUN			

SHOPPING LIST

WEEK 9: FOOD JOURNAL

Day 1

DATE:

BREAKFAST: carbs:

LUNCH: carbs:

DINNER: carbs:

SNACKS: carbs:

WATER INTAKE:

WEEK 9: FOOD JOURNAL

Day 2

DATE:

BREAKFAST: *carbs:*

LUNCH: *carbs:*

DINNER: *carbs:*

SNACKS: *carbs:*

WATER INTAKE:

WEEK 9: FOOD JOURNAL

Day 3

DATE:

BREAKFAST: *carbs:*

LUNCH: *carbs:*

DINNER: *carbs:*

SNACKS: *carbs:*

WATER INTAKE:

WEEK 9: FOOD JOURNAL

Day 4

DATE:

BREAKFAST: carbs:

LUNCH: carbs:

DINNER: carbs:

SNACKS: carbs:

WATER INTAKE:

WEEK 9: FOOD JOURNAL

Day 5

DATE:

BREAKFAST: carbs:

LUNCH: carbs:

DINNER: carbs:

SNACKS: carbs:

WATER INTAKE:

WEEK 9: FOOD JOURNAL

Day 6

DATE:

BREAKFAST: carbs:

LUNCH: carbs:

DINNER: carbs:

SNACKS: carbs:

WATER INTAKE:

WEEK 9: FOOD JOURNAL

Day 7

DATE:

BREAKFAST: carbs:

LUNCH: carbs:

DINNER: carbs:

SNACKS: carbs:

WATER INTAKE:

WEEK 9: RESULTS

DATE:

	MEASUREMENT:	LOSS/GAIN:
WEIGHT:		
LEFT ARM:		
RIGHT ARM:		
CHEST:		
WAIST:		
HIPS:		
LEFT THIGH:		
RIGHT THIGH:		

Weekly Goals

WEEK 10: SELF-CARE

DATE

SELF CARE CHECKLIST:

- [ ]
- [ ]
- [ ]
- [ ]
- [ ]
- [ ]
- [ ]
- [ ]
- [ ]
- [ ]

FOCUS FOR THE WEEK:

WHAT MOTIVATES ME:

SELF CARE CHECKLIST

GOALS	M	T	W	T	F	S	S
Got enough rest	○	○	○	○	○	○	○
Drank water	○	○	○	○	○	○	○
Exercised	○	○	○	○	○	○	○
Ate Mindfully	○	○	○	○	○	○	○
____________	○	○	○	○	○	○	○
____________	○	○	○	○	○	○	○
____________	○	○	○	○	○	○	○
____________	○	○	○	○	○	○	○
____________	○	○	○	○	○	○	○
____________	○	○	○	○	○	○	○
____________	○	○	○	○	○	○	○

WEEK 10: OVERVIEW

DAILY PLAN
MON:
TUES:
WED:
THUR:
FRI:
SAT:
SUN:

TO DO LIST:

- [ ]
- [ ]
- [ ]
- [ ]
- [ ]
- [ ]
- [ ]
- [ ]
- [ ]
- [ ]

NOTES & REMINDERS

THOUGHTS

WEEK 10: TOP 3 GOALS

GOAL	STEPS TO MAKE IT HAPPEN	DATE	✓

GOAL	STEPS TO MAKE IT HAPPEN	DATE	✓

GOAL	STEPS TO MAKE IT HAPPEN	DATE	✓

WEEK 10: EXERCISE

MON	
TUE	
WED	
THUR	
FRI	
SAT	
SUN	

INTERMITTENT FASTING *Tracker*

WEEK OF:

Monday																								
Goal	12	1	2	3	4	5	6	7	8	9	10	11	12	1	2	3	4	5	6	7	8	9	10	11
Actual	12	1	2	3	4	5	6	7	8	9	10	11	12	1	2	3	4	5	6	7	8	9	10	11

Tuesday																								
Goal	12	1	2	3	4	5	6	7	8	9	10	11	12	1	2	3	4	5	6	7	8	9	10	11
Actual	12	1	2	3	4	5	6	7	8	9	10	11	12	1	2	3	4	5	6	7	8	9	10	11

Wednesday																								
Goal	12	1	2	3	4	5	6	7	8	9	10	11	12	1	2	3	4	5	6	7	8	9	10	11
Actual	12	1	2	3	4	5	6	7	8	9	10	11	12	1	2	3	4	5	6	7	8	9	10	11

Thursday																								
Goal	12	1	2	3	4	5	6	7	8	9	10	11	12	1	2	3	4	5	6	7	8	9	10	11
Actual	12	1	2	3	4	5	6	7	8	9	10	11	12	1	2	3	4	5	6	7	8	9	10	11

Friday																								
Goal	12	1	2	3	4	5	6	7	8	9	10	11	12	1	2	3	4	5	6	7	8	9	10	11
Actual	12	1	2	3	4	5	6	7	8	9	10	11	12	1	2	3	4	5	6	7	8	9	10	11

Saturday																								
Goal	12	1	2	3	4	5	6	7	8	9	10	11	12	1	2	3	4	5	6	7	8	9	10	11
Actual	12	1	2	3	4	5	6	7	8	9	10	11	12	1	2	3	4	5	6	7	8	9	10	11

Sunday																								
Goal	12	1	2	3	4	5	6	7	8	9	10	11	12	1	2	3	4	5	6	7	8	9	10	11
Actual	12	1	2	3	4	5	6	7	8	9	10	11	12	1	2	3	4	5	6	7	8	9	10	11

WEEK 10: MEAL PLANS

	BREAKFAST	LUNCH	DINNER
MON			
TUES			
WED			
THU			
FRI			
SAT			
SUN			

SHOPPING LIST

WEEK 10: FOOD JOURNAL

Day 1

DATE:

BREAKFAST: carbs:

LUNCH: carbs:

DINNER: carbs:

SNACKS: carbs:

WATER INTAKE:

WEEK 10: FOOD JOURNAL

Day 2

DATE:

BREAKFAST: carbs:

LUNCH: carbs:

DINNER: carbs:

SNACKS: carbs:

WATER INTAKE:

WEEK 10: FOOD JOURNAL

Day 3

DATE:

BREAKFAST: carbs:

LUNCH: carbs:

DINNER: carbs:

SNACKS: carbs:

WATER INTAKE:

WEEK 10: FOOD JOURNAL

Day 4

DATE:

BREAKFAST: carbs:

LUNCH: carbs:

DINNER: carbs:

SNACKS: carbs:

WATER INTAKE:

WEEK 10: FOOD JOURNAL

Day 5

DATE:

BREAKFAST: carbs:

LUNCH: carbs:

DINNER: carbs:

SNACKS: carbs:

WATER INTAKE:

WEEK 10: FOOD JOURNAL

Day 6

DATE:

BREAKFAST: carbs:

LUNCH: carbs:

DINNER: carbs:

SNACKS: carbs:

WATER INTAKE:

WEEK 10: FOOD JOURNAL

Day 7

DATE:

BREAKFAST: *carbs:*

LUNCH: *carbs:*

DINNER: *carbs:*

SNACKS: *carbs:*

WATER INTAKE:

WEEK 10: RESULTS

DATE:

	MEASUREMENT:	LOSS/GAIN:
WEIGHT:		
LEFT ARM:		
RIGHT ARM:		
CHEST:		
WAIST:		
HIPS:		
LEFT THIGH:		
RIGHT THIGH:		

Weekly Goals

WEEK 11: SELF-CARE

DATE

SELF CARE CHECKLIST:

FOCUS FOR THE WEEK:

WHAT MOTIVATES ME:

SELF CARE CHECKLIST

GOALS	M	T	W	T	F	S	S
Got enough rest	○	○	○	○	○	○	○
Drank water	○	○	○	○	○	○	○
Exercised	○	○	○	○	○	○	○
Ate Mindfully	○	○	○	○	○	○	○
____________	○	○	○	○	○	○	○
____________	○	○	○	○	○	○	○
____________	○	○	○	○	○	○	○
____________	○	○	○	○	○	○	○
____________	○	○	○	○	○	○	○
____________	○	○	○	○	○	○	○
____________	○	○	○	○	○	○	○

WEEK 11: OVERVIEW

DAILY PLAN
MON:
TUES:
WED:
THUR:
FRI:
SAT:
SUN:

TO DO LIST:

- [ ]
- [ ]
- [ ]
- [ ]
- [ ]
- [ ]
- [ ]
- [ ]
- [ ]
- [ ]

NOTES & REMINDERS

THOUGHTS

WEEK 11: TOP 3 GOALS

GOAL	STEPS TO MAKE IT HAPPEN	DATE	✓

GOAL	STEPS TO MAKE IT HAPPEN	DATE	✓

GOAL	STEPS TO MAKE IT HAPPEN	DATE	✓

WEEK 11: EXERCISE

MON	
TUE	
WED	
THUR	
FRI	
SAT	
SUN	

INTERMITTENT FASTING *Tracker*

WEEK OF:

Monday																								
Goal	12	1	2	3	4	5	6	7	8	9	10	11	12	1	2	3	4	5	6	7	8	9	10	11
Actual	12	1	2	3	4	5	6	7	8	9	10	11	12	1	2	3	4	5	6	7	8	9	10	11

Tuesday																								
Goal	12	1	2	3	4	5	6	7	8	9	10	11	12	1	2	3	4	5	6	7	8	9	10	11
Actual	12	1	2	3	4	5	6	7	8	9	10	11	12	1	2	3	4	5	6	7	8	9	10	11

Wednesday																								
Goal	12	1	2	3	4	5	6	7	8	9	10	11	12	1	2	3	4	5	6	7	8	9	10	11
Actual	12	1	2	3	4	5	6	7	8	9	10	11	12	1	2	3	4	5	6	7	8	9	10	11

Thursday																								
Goal	12	1	2	3	4	5	6	7	8	9	10	11	12	1	2	3	4	5	6	7	8	9	10	11
Actual	12	1	2	3	4	5	6	7	8	9	10	11	12	1	2	3	4	5	6	7	8	9	10	11

Friday																								
Goal	12	1	2	3	4	5	6	7	8	9	10	11	12	1	2	3	4	5	6	7	8	9	10	11
Actual	12	1	2	3	4	5	6	7	8	9	10	11	12	1	2	3	4	5	6	7	8	9	10	11

Saturday																								
Goal	12	1	2	3	4	5	6	7	8	9	10	11	12	1	2	3	4	5	6	7	8	9	10	11
Actual	12	1	2	3	4	5	6	7	8	9	10	11	12	1	2	3	4	5	6	7	8	9	10	11

Sunday																								
Goal	12	1	2	3	4	5	6	7	8	9	10	11	12	1	2	3	4	5	6	7	8	9	10	11
Actual	12	1	2	3	4	5	6	7	8	9	10	11	12	1	2	3	4	5	6	7	8	9	10	11

WEEK 11: MEAL PLANS

	BREAKFAST	LUNCH	DINNER
MON			
TUES			
WED			
THU			
FRI			
SAT			
SUN			

SHOPPING LIST

WEEK 11: FOOD JOURNAL

Day 1

DATE:

BREAKFAST: *carbs:*

LUNCH: *carbs:*

DINNER: *carbs:*

SNACKS: *carbs:*

WATER INTAKE:

WEEK 11: FOOD JOURNAL

Day 2

DATE:

BREAKFAST: *carbs:*

LUNCH: *carbs:*

DINNER: *carbs:*

SNACKS: *carbs:*

WATER INTAKE:

WEEK 11: FOOD JOURNAL

Day 3

DATE:

BREAKFAST: carbs:

LUNCH: carbs:

DINNER: carbs:

SNACKS: carbs:

WATER INTAKE:

WEEK 11: FOOD JOURNAL

Day 4

DATE:

BREAKFAST: *carbs:*

LUNCH: *carbs:*

DINNER: *carbs:*

SNACKS: *carbs:*

WATER INTAKE:

WEEK 11: FOOD JOURNAL

Day 5

DATE:

BREAKFAST: carbs:

LUNCH: carbs:

DINNER: carbs:

SNACKS: carbs:

WATER INTAKE:

WEEK 11: FOOD JOURNAL

Day 6

DATE:

BREAKFAST: carbs:

LUNCH: carbs:

DINNER: carbs:

SNACKS: carbs:

WATER INTAKE:

WEEK 11: FOOD JOURNAL

Day 7

DATE:

BREAKFAST: carbs:

LUNCH: carbs:

DINNER: carbs:

SNACKS: carbs:

WATER INTAKE:

WEEK 11: RESULTS

DATE:

	MEASUREMENT:	LOSS/GAIN:
WEIGHT:		
LEFT ARM:		
RIGHT ARM:		
CHEST:		
WAIST:		
HIPS:		
LEFT THIGH:		
RIGHT THIGH:		

Weekly Goals

WEEK 12: SELF-CARE

DATE

SELF CARE CHECKLIST:

FOCUS FOR THE WEEK:

WHAT MOTIVATES ME:

SELF CARE CHECKLIST

GOALS	M	T	W	T	F	S	S
Got enough rest	○	○	○	○	○	○	○
Drank water	○	○	○	○	○	○	○
Exercised	○	○	○	○	○	○	○
Ate Mindfully	○	○	○	○	○	○	○
________________	○	○	○	○	○	○	○
________________	○	○	○	○	○	○	○
________________	○	○	○	○	○	○	○
________________	○	○	○	○	○	○	○
________________	○	○	○	○	○	○	○
________________	○	○	○	○	○	○	○
________________	○	○	○	○	○	○	○

WEEK 12: OVERVIEW

DAILY PLAN
MON:
TUES:
WED:
THUR:
FRI:
SAT:
SUN:

TO DO LIST:

NOTES & REMINDERS

THOUGHTS

WEEK 12: TOP 3 GOALS

GOAL	STEPS TO MAKE IT HAPPEN	DATE	✓

GOAL	STEPS TO MAKE IT HAPPEN	DATE	✓

GOAL	STEPS TO MAKE IT HAPPEN	DATE	✓

WEEK 12: EXERCISE

MON	
TUE	
WED	
THUR	
FRI	
SAT	
SUN	

INTERMITTENT FASTING *Tracker*

WEEK OF:

Monday																								
Goal	12	1	2	3	4	5	6	7	8	9	10	11	12	1	2	3	4	5	6	7	8	9	10	11
Actual	12	1	2	3	4	5	6	7	8	9	10	11	12	1	2	3	4	5	6	7	8	9	10	11

Tuesday																								
Goal	12	1	2	3	4	5	6	7	8	9	10	11	12	1	2	3	4	5	6	7	8	9	10	11
Actual	12	1	2	3	4	5	6	7	8	9	10	11	12	1	2	3	4	5	6	7	8	9	10	11

Wednesday																								
Goal	12	1	2	3	4	5	6	7	8	9	10	11	12	1	2	3	4	5	6	7	8	9	10	11
Actual	12	1	2	3	4	5	6	7	8	9	10	11	12	1	2	3	4	5	6	7	8	9	10	11

Thursday																								
Goal	12	1	2	3	4	5	6	7	8	9	10	11	12	1	2	3	4	5	6	7	8	9	10	11
Actual	12	1	2	3	4	5	6	7	8	9	10	11	12	1	2	3	4	5	6	7	8	9	10	11

Friday																								
Goal	12	1	2	3	4	5	6	7	8	9	10	11	12	1	2	3	4	5	6	7	8	9	10	11
Actual	12	1	2	3	4	5	6	7	8	9	10	11	12	1	2	3	4	5	6	7	8	9	10	11

Saturday																								
Goal	12	1	2	3	4	5	6	7	8	9	10	11	12	1	2	3	4	5	6	7	8	9	10	11
Actual	12	1	2	3	4	5	6	7	8	9	10	11	12	1	2	3	4	5	6	7	8	9	10	11

Sunday																								
Goal	12	1	2	3	4	5	6	7	8	9	10	11	12	1	2	3	4	5	6	7	8	9	10	11
Actual	12	1	2	3	4	5	6	7	8	9	10	11	12	1	2	3	4	5	6	7	8	9	10	11

WEEK 12: MEAL PLANS

	BREAKFAST	LUNCH	DINNER
MON			
TUES			
WED			
THU			
FRI			
SAT			
SUN			

SHOPPING LIST

WEEK 12: FOOD JOURNAL

Day 1

DATE:

BREAKFAST: carbs:

LUNCH: carbs:

DINNER: carbs:

SNACKS: carbs:

WATER INTAKE:

WEEK 12: FOOD JOURNAL

Day 2

DATE:

BREAKFAST: *carbs:*

LUNCH: *carbs:*

DINNER: *carbs:*

SNACKS: *carbs:*

WATER INTAKE:

WEEK 12: FOOD JOURNAL

Day 3

DATE:

BREAKFAST: *carbs:*

LUNCH: *carbs:*

DINNER: *carbs:*

SNACKS: *carbs:*

WATER INTAKE:

WEEK 12: FOOD JOURNAL

Day 4

DATE:

BREAKFAST: carbs:

LUNCH: carbs:

DINNER: carbs:

SNACKS: carbs:

WATER INTAKE:

WEEK 12: FOOD JOURNAL

Day 5

DATE:

BREAKFAST: carbs:

LUNCH: carbs:

DINNER: carbs:

SNACKS: carbs:

WATER INTAKE:

WEEK 12: FOOD JOURNAL

Day 6

DATE:

BREAKFAST: carbs:

LUNCH: carbs:

DINNER: carbs:

SNACKS: carbs:

WATER INTAKE:

WEEK 12: FOOD JOURNAL

Day 7

DATE:

BREAKFAST: *carbs:*

LUNCH: *carbs:*

DINNER: *carbs:*

SNACKS: *carbs:*

WATER INTAKE:

WEEK 12: RESULTS

DATE:

	MEASUREMENT:	LOSS/GAIN:
WEIGHT:		
LEFT ARM:		
RIGHT ARM:		
CHEST:		
WAIST:		
HIPS:		
LEFT THIGH:		
RIGHT THIGH:		

Weekly Goals

GOALS

WHEN	MY GOALS	STEPS
6 MONTHS		
1 YEAR		
2 YEARS		
5 YEARS		

INSPIRATION

WHAT I LEARNED:

Made in the USA
Las Vegas, NV
16 February 2024